# STORIES OF SURVIVAL

AMY WONG

# STORIES
# OF SURVIVAL

The Paradox of Suicide Vulnerability
and Resiliency among Asian American
College Students

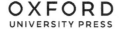

OXFORD
UNIVERSITY PRESS

# OXFORD
## UNIVERSITY PRESS

Oxford University Press is a department of the University of Oxford. It furthers
the University's objective of excellence in research, scholarship, and education
by publishing worldwide. Oxford is a registered trade mark of Oxford University
Press in the UK and certain other countries.

Published in the United States of America by Oxford University Press
198 Madison Avenue, New York, NY 10016, United States of America.

Library of Congress Cataloging-in-Publication Data
Names: Wong, Amy, 1965– author.
Title: Stories of survival : the paradox of suicide vulnerability and
resiliency among Asian American college students / Amy Wong.
Other titles: Paradox of suicide vulnerability and resiliency among Asian
American college students
Description: New York, NY : Oxford University Press, [2023] |
Includes bibliographical references and index.
Identifiers: LCCN 2023006231 (print) | LCCN 2023006232 (ebook) |
ISBN 9780197662397 (paperback) | ISBN 9780197662410 (epub) | ISBN 9780197662427
Subjects: MESH: Suicidal Ideation | Resilience, Psychological | Risk
Factors | Students—psychology | Universities | Asian | United States
Classification: LCC RC569 (print) | LCC RC569 (ebook) | NLM WM 165 |
DDC 616.85/844500835—dc23/eng/20230302
LC record available at https://lccn.loc.gov/2023006231
LC ebook record available at https://lccn.loc.gov/2023006232

DOI: 10.1093/oso/9780197662397.001.0001

This material is not intended to be, and should not be considered, a substitute for medical or other
professional advice. Treatment for the conditions described in this material is highly dependent on
the individual circumstances. And, while this material is designed to offer accurate information with
respect to the subject matter covered and to be current as of the time it was written, research and
knowledge about medical and health issues is constantly evolving and dose schedules for medications
are being revised continually, with new side effects recognized and accounted for regularly. Readers
must therefore always check the product information and clinical procedures with the most up-to-date
published product information and data sheets provided by the manufacturers and the most recent
codes of conduct and safety regulation. The publisher and the authors make no representations or
warranties to readers, express or implied, as to the accuracy or completeness of this material. Without
limiting the foregoing, the publisher and the authors make no representations or warranties as to the
accuracy or efficacy of the drug dosages mentioned in the material. The authors and the publisher do
not accept, and expressly disclaim, any responsibility for any liability, loss, or risk that may be claimed
or incurred as a consequence of the use and/or application of any of the contents of this material.

Printed by Marquis Book Printing, Canada

This book is dedicated to anyone who has been touched by suicide ideation, suicidal behaviors, and suicide deaths.

I believe that one of the most important missions of sociology is to give voice—to give voice to the experiences of those whose voices and experiences would typically otherwise be blunted, marginalized, shifted off to the side or simply ignored. If we want to understand how society works, if we want to understand how social structures structure us, we need particularly to listen well to the narratives of those who are too often powerless, marginalized, disenfranchised, and stigmatized.

David A. Karp
*Voices from the Inside: Readings on the Experiences of Mental Illness* (2010, p. 4)

How stories are told, who tells them, when they're told, how many stories are told—are really dependent on power.

Chimamanda Ngozi Adichie
*The Danger of a Single Story*
TED Talk, October 2009

# CONTENTS

*Preface*                                                                ix
*Acknowledgments*                                                      xvii

Introduction                                                              1
  Suicides in the United States                                 5
  Asian Americans                                               6
  The Paradox of Vulnerability and Resiliency                   8
  Risk Factors and Vulnerability                               18
  Protective Factors and Resiliency                            23
  A Collection of Human Stories                                29

1. The Risk Factors for Suicide Ideation                                 33
  History of Mental Health Challenges                          34
  "Today Is a Bad Day"                                         40
  Intergenerational Trauma                                     46
  Thwarted Belongingness                                       51
  Perceived Burdensomeness                                     71

2. The Protective Factors Against Suicide Death                          91
  The Global Pandemic                                          93
  Coping Strategies and Self-Reliance                         103
  Support Systems and Human Attachment                        112
  Life Skills and Self-Care                                   121
  "Today Is a Good Day"                                       130
  Reasons for Living                                          135

3. Addressing the Paradox of Suicide Vulnerability and
   Resiliency                                                      144
   Understanding Vulnerability and Reducing Risk Factors      147
   Understanding Resiliency and Promoting Protective
       Factors                                                    161
   The Call for Action                                            170
   Practice Recommendations                                       172
   Research Recommendations                                       191
   Conclusion                                                     193

*Afterword*                                                        195
*Notes*                                                            201
*Index*                                                            221

# PREFACE

I was inspired to write this book for several different reasons. First, I had been teaching in higher education for more than 25 years when I recently decided to continue my studies to earn a doctoral degree. This more current educational journey profoundly shaped my research direction. As I progressed in my studies, I was challenged to consider a problem of practice that would address an institutional concern negatively impacting the student population. More important, I was advised that this problem of practice should be professionally significant, academically challenging, and personally meaningful. Although I was interested in several investigative prospects, including campus racism, free speech in the classroom, and teaching controversial subject matters, I ultimately focused on college suicidal ideation and behaviors. The decision to choose this particular subject matter was greatly influenced by the second major experience in my professional life as a faculty member.

Working as a faculty member means that I am in constant contact with students in my lecture halls and campus office. In the classrooms, we cover an array of general topics in sociology, such as current events pertaining to social class, race and ethnicity, and sex and gender. More specific lectures focus on food insecurity and homelessness, police brutality and hate crimes, or intimate partner violence and rape culture. According to my students throughout the years, the lectures on the sociology of the body—particularly the mental health aspects—were well received and greatly appreciated. To introduce this important subject matter, I provide an overview on mental health and then focus specifically on major depressive disorder and its connections to suicide ideation and suicide deaths. As students of sociology, we examine the external and social factors that may contribute to aggravating psychological vulnerabilities. Students are generally more engaged in these class discussions. In some of my teaching evaluations, students identify these topics as their favorite lectures because they are personally relevant and meaningful. In my own teaching reflections, I noted that students tend to be more engaged in their studies if they have a personal connection to the subject matter. I found that the merging of their individual experiences with mental health difficulties and developing scholarship on major depressive disorder provided the foundation for our continuing conversations. It was during office hours with students that I further understood the significance of the mental health literature to their personal lives.

One of my teaching joys is getting to know my students better. I like learning about their backgrounds and understanding why they have chosen this particular university to work on a specific major. Sometimes my students talk about their diverse academic interests in the social sciences and how they imagine their futures will unfold. The college years are such an exciting time for them to explore and develop their full potential. They ask a lot questions about my own experiences as a former student of political science, sociology, and education; moreover, they want to know what it means to be a sociologist. These exchanges of academic and professional information between the students and me are some of my favorite responsibilities as a teacher. During these office meetings, the students usually engage in more personal sharing about their feelings and emotions. We talk about academic stress and competition. We talk about the difficult and challenging work that comes with earning a university degree. There are concerns about choosing the right classes for the right major for the right job market. Students speak about roommate challenges and financial constraints. In general, students openly express their stress and anxiety during our meetings. Students understand I am not trained to diagnose them, and perhaps this encourages them to be more open and honest with me. Rather, it is my responsibility to listen to their concerns and offer human kindness. It is also my practice to guide them to further readings and to recommend campus resources.

In the many years of listening to students, my own interest about mental health concerns continued to grow. My long history of working with college students showed a shift in our office conversations regarding personal suffering. In the past few years, I found that students were more willing to talk about their mental health troubles. When I first started my teaching career, the topic of mental health distress did not usually come to the surface. Witnessing the shift, I started to wonder if students were more mentally vulnerable now than they were 20-odd years ago or if I was working with a new generation that was more aware of their feelings and more open to discussing them with their college professors. It is also possible that there is now more available information about general mental health and this has created more social awareness and acceptance about individual vulnerability. I have come to understand that college students experience psychological stress as they work toward their college degrees. Furthermore, it is not a social phenomenon that will soon go away.

I have made it my goal to acquire more information about college students and overall mental health. The university website was a productive place to learn about available campus resources, and I read with great interest the entire section dedicated to faculty who worked with psychologically distressed students. This early information also served the purpose of allowing me to be a better resource and advocate for my students. It was with this personal desire for more knowledge and a strong sense of professional development that I was able to move in a particular direction with my dissertation. I had found a problem of practice that was professionally significant, academically challenging, and personally meaningful. I continued my investigation on college students who have experienced psychological suffering, and this process led me to focus on Asian American college students who have experienced suicide ideation.

As a mostly teaching sociologist, I was aware of my limitations. I did not have an academic background in psychology or psychiatry. However, my training in the social sciences facilitated the research process. The literature review took me to suicide ideation, suicidal tendencies, and college suicides. I learned that some college student subgroups were more vulnerable to suicide ideation, suicidal behaviors, and suicide deaths. These identified student subgroups came mostly from marginalized populations, including the African American, transgender, and Asian American communities. I also noted that these student subgroups were framed around a deficit-based perspective. These studies focused on the weaknesses of these student subgroups by highlighting their experiences with marginalization, discrimination, and racism.

The research on suicide ideation from a strength-based perspective was more difficult to find. I did not review as many articles about a college student's strength, resolve, or resiliency against depression or suicide ideation. In my mind, this did not make sense because clearly not all depressed or suicidal individuals die by suicide. I wondered about their experiences and considered how they managed their lives as suicidal college students. More important, I was not hearing the voices of people who experienced suicidal ideation or behavior in the research. It was a bit troubling to understand one of the most painful experiences a person could go through reduced to a few numbers in a quantitative study. The literature review process revealed reams of numerical data, but a fair amount of missing descriptive and explanatory data. On the one hand, I understood the need to have numerical data in order to demonstrate that suicide ideation is a social problem. Indeed, the numbers told me that too many people consider suicide each year. On the other hand, the numbers did not humanize the individuals' experiences with suicide ideation. The numbers did not help me understand the magnitude of a person's suffering and pain. What did a suicidal individual feel? How would they describe their distress? When did they have suicidal thoughts? I wanted to hear in their own words how they would describe and explain their journey into mental suffering and pain. More important, I wanted to understand how they survived while living with suicide ideation.

The third event that informed the contents of this book was the development of the global pandemic. By this time, I had already decided to focus on Asian American college students and their experiences with suicide ideation. As I continued to develop my research project within the context of the emerging global pandemic, I wondered if anyone would be willing to spend the time to talk with me. As universities throughout the nation started sending students to virtual classrooms, would any students accept an invitation to participate in yet another virtual conversation, especially to talk about something that was deeply personal and painful? In addition, there was a general fear of living as an Asian American person in the United States, especially as Asians and Asian Americans were blamed for the origins of the coronavirus and anti-Asian hate crimes were on the rise. I was concerned that students would not want to share their private anguish and torment with a researcher during this intensified time of violence directed against individuals who were perceived as Asian. I felt my work as a researcher would be viewed with trepidation and exhaustion. Yet, at the same time, I felt that reaching out to Asian American college students to hear their stories about psychological distress within the context of COVID-19 took on a greater urgency; if anything, the pandemic strengthened my determination to try. In the end, I did find Asian American college students who were willing to share their stories with me. I credit my positionality and identity as a Chinese American researcher in helping me reach potential participants.

The student interviews took place from fall 2020 to spring 2021 when the world was living through the first year of the global pandemic. In light of this developing social climate, I added an interview question about the global pandemic. It was not my intention to think about comparative work regarding what students experienced before the pandemic and what they experienced after; rather, I wanted to hear their stories about psychological distress in any way that they wanted to share them with me. It was also a bit early for college students to think about before and after when they were living in the here and now of the pandemic, struggling to keep it all together. On many levels, this was a time that was ripe for potential participants to share their stories. Asian American college students already demonstrated high rates of suicide ideation, and the ongoing pandemic intensified these existing suicidal tendencies and behaviors. In an academic year, I was able to interview 12 college students who were willing to talk with me about their mental health challenges before and during the global pandemic.

The purpose of this book is to reach a wide audience about suicide ideation and suicide resiliency in the United States. In my opinion, we do not talk enough about mental health challenges. I would like us to be a more open society willing to engage in meaningful and constructive conversations that matter to human beings. It is the goal of this book to reduce the stigma, shame, and silence associated with mental health difficulties. In short, I hope this book begins or continues the conversations about suicide ideation, suicidal behaviors, and suicide deaths. With deep appreciation, I found that Asian American college students were willing to talk with me about their experiences with suicide ideation. Ultimately, their willingness to speak openly and authentically about their mental health struggles made the contents of this book possible.

# ACKNOWLEDGMENTS

This book evolved from my dissertation work at the USC Rossier School of Education. I appreciate the dedication of my chair, Patricia Tobey, and committee members, Monique Datta and Derisa Grant. They encouraged me to rework my chapters as a book to ensure that this subject matter reached a wider audience. I am deeply grateful for their academic guidance and professional support. Other professors inspired me along the way. Courtney Malloy, Maria Ott, and Raquel Torres-Retana challenged me to think about my own work in higher education as a researcher, teacher, and agent of change. I am thankful for our robust classroom conversations.

The Department of Sociology at San Diego State University has been my professional home for many years. It is an understatement to say that my colleagues and I are usually busy with our teaching schedules and writing projects. While we remain committed to our work, it is a nice surprise when we are able to talk for more than a few minutes. The informal chats we have in the halls or meeting for coffee one building over are meaningful expressions of good will and department collegiality. I appreciate the friendships I have cultivated in this special space. I love being a faculty member here and enjoy working with my colleagues.

I am deeply grateful for my editor at Oxford University Press, Sarah Humphreville, who saw the potential in this book during the early stages. She encouraged me to use my voice to authentically write this book. Our meetings were always productive, and I appreciate all the support and advice she gave me. I also give a lot of credit to my project editor, Emma Hodgdon, for helping me envision the final production of my book. She helped me think about potential book covers and formatting styles. Finally, I thank the anonymous readers who reviewed my book proposal and offered constructive insights.

I am sincerely thankful for all the willing college students who shared their stories with me. Their powerful words allowed me to write this book with clarity, purpose, and conviction.

There are lovely people who are part of my beloved community. I have known these individuals my whole life or most of my life. I know I can count on them for encouragement and companionship. These loved ones have embraced me for a long time, and I am genuinely appreciative for their presence in my life.

This book begins and ends with my own family. I found the courage and endurance in writing this book because I had two people in my corner who cared about me. I am profoundly grateful for Dwayne and Shel for bringing light, love, and joy to my world.

# INTRODUCTION

This book is a collection of narratives about human survival. It tells the stories of individuals who have experienced suicide ideation and how they have managed to stay alive. Because this book is about endurance, it is also about courage and hope. These individuals have shown that they have the courage to hope for the promise of a new day. In sharing their experiences with me, they are communicating their particular vulnerabilities to suicide ideation and their specific resiliencies to suicide death. In this way, they are addressing the risk factors of suicide ideation while also expressing the protective factors that prevent suicide death. Although this book focuses on Asian American college students, it is not just for Asian Americans or college students. It is for all of us who identify with stories of human vulnerability and resiliency.

This book is written for several audiences in mind. First, it is for all of us who have been touched by suicide ideation and suicide deaths. In these stories, we might see a bit of our own life experiences which will help us to understand that we are not alone in our personal struggles. It may also be meaningful to readers to recognize that suffering and pain are universal human experiences. We all have our own stories of sorrow and grief. At the same time, the journey in life often includes our resolve,

*Stories of Survival.* Amy Wong, Oxford University Press. © Oxford University Press 2023.
DOI: 10.1093/oso/9780197662397.003.0001

strength, and resiliency. Accordingly, we have our stories of happiness and joy. These college students have articulated some of their most challenging moments and how they managed to get through the day, week, month, and year. In some of the most distressing points in their lives, they also found the ability to handle their negative thoughts and emotions. Over and over again, these individuals also experienced contentment and gratification. On the whole, these students shared their stories of determination with me. I hope that this book will be a source of inspiration for all of us who hope to live a full life.

Second, it is for the general reader who has a curiosity for human stories and current events. At the time of this writing, there has been a steady flow of news reports on Asian Americans, the global pandemic, and mental health distress; therefore, this book may appeal to individuals who want to learn more about these three interconnected topics. This book also stands alone to give voice to Asian American college students who have lived with—and managed—psychological pain throughout the years. This book is relevant now and will be in the years to come for people who want to learn more about the pandemic's impact on one segment of the U.S. population. Although there is a growing body of suicide scholarship found in academic journals and readers, there are fewer accessible books to the general reader. Therefore, it was one of my goals to bring the suicide research where it usually resides in the academy to a more general audience.

Third, this book is for all college and university stakeholders, including students, faculty, and administrators. Even before the pandemic, college students had been experiencing an increase in mental health challenges and difficulties, including anxiety, depression, and suicide ideation. In general, there has been a collective concern about college students as they navigate their higher education years away from home and deal with personal, social, and educational obstacles. There remains a growing interest—and alarm—for the college population and their mental well-being before, during, and after the global pandemic. This book gives voice to the college experience that is not always ideal. Going to college and earning a bachelor's degree are already difficult and challenging goals. For individuals who live with depression and suicide ideation, the educational journey is much more difficult. College personnel should be made aware of these challenges and difficulties. Furthermore, this book offers several practice recommendations to college personnel as they continue to work with vulnerable student populations.

Fourth, mental health practitioners and researchers may find the information in this book applicable and useful in their own professional work. For example, counselors and therapists may be able to use the information from this book to work more productivity with the student population seeking professional mental health services. In addition, mental health researchers may use the information from this book to develop different research directions in the broad areas of suicide ideation and suicide deaths. The important and robust work continues for mental health counselors and researchers as they engage and work with diverse student populations. It is important to note that Asian American college students may have different and specific needs with regard to understanding and utilizing mental health services. Furthermore, counseling offices may want to consider how they can reach different segments of the college population so that they receive mental health resources and services.

Finally, organizations that focus on suicide prevention may find the information in this book as a productive resource in their own advocacy work. Organizations such as the American Association of Suicidology, American Foundation for Suicide Prevention, JED Foundation, Suicide Prevention Resource Center, and Higher Education Mental Health Alliance may be able to use the information in this book to advance their own suicide prevention programs. These organizations collect suicide scholarship and work diligently to share resources in order to address the social problem of suicides in the United States.

Before going further, the language we use to explain the experiences of a suicidal person is an important consideration. The National Institute of Mental Health provides the following language to help individuals understand the meaning of suicide, suicide attempt, and suicidal ideation. *Suicide* is death caused by self-directed injurious behavior with the intent to die as a result of the behavior. *Suicide attempt* is a nonfatal, self-directed, potentially injurious behavior with the intent to die as a result of the behavior; a suicide attempt might not result in injury. *Suicidal ideation* is thinking about, considering, or planning suicide.[1] Having this vocabulary allows individuals, families, and other loved ones to frame an understanding that thoughts, planning, and action are connected to the experiences of a suicidal person.

Some common terms we have used to talk about suicide include "committed suicide," "successful suicide," "failed suicide attempt," or "completed suicide." These phrases have been so repeatedly used that we often do not question the specific word choices. However, it may be more considerate to use neutral words to describe the act of suicide.[2] The word "commit" has criminal overtones that refer to a past time when it was illegal to kill oneself; committing suicide

4

was synonymous with committing murder. Similarly, it is difficult to try to frame the act of suicide in a positive way by calling it a "successful suicide" or to further evaluate a horrible experience as a "failed suicide attempt." Death by suicide does not need the added adjective of being a "completed suicide." In writing this book, I have chosen to use more impartial language: death by suicide, nonfatal suicide attempt, died by suicide, suicide, and suicide death. The carefully chosen words we use to talk about self-harm help us develop a more compassionate understanding of suicide.

## Suicides in the United States

Suicide is a leading cause of death in the United States. According to the Centers for Disease Control and Prevention, suicide rates increased 30% between 2000 and 2018 and declined in 2019 and 2020.[3] There were 45,979 suicide deaths in 2020, which is approximately one death every 11 minutes. On average, there are 130 suicides per day.[4] These numbers tell us that suicide deaths are a social phenomenon in the United States. As we bring our focus to the specific population of college students, the numbers remain troubling.

College suicides are a social problem in the United States. The research data show that young adults are at risk for suicide ideation and suicide deaths. For example, suicide is the second leading cause of death among 18- to 24-year-old adults,[5] and it is estimated that 1,088 college students die by suicide each year in the United States.[6] The American College Health Association surveyed 26,685 students and found that 6.4% had seriously considered suicide and 1.3% had attempted suicide in the prior 12 months.[7] Similarly, more than half of all college students experienced some level of suicide ideation in their lifetime.[8] As I continued to delve more into the suicide scholarship, I also learned more about the history of Asian Americans and Asian American college students.

## Asian Americans

Asian Americans include a diversity of ethnic groups that have a long history in the United States. The early arrival of different Asian groups to the United States included the Chinese, Filipino, Indian, Japanese, Korean, and Vietnamese peoples.[9] In 2019, these six origin groups made up 85% of all Asian Americans. Figure I.1

**Six origin groups make up 85% of all Asian Americans**

*% of the U.S. Asian population that is...*

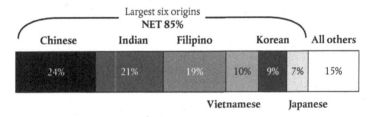

Note: "All others" includes the 3% of U.S. Asians in the category "Other Asian, not specified." "Chinese" includes those identifying as Taiwanese. For more about measuring the Taiwanese population in the U.S., read "How many Taiwanese live in the U.S.? It's not an easy question to answer." Figures do not add to 100% because individuals identifying with more than one Asian group are included in all groups. Figure for all origin groups includes mixed-race and mixed-group populations, regardless of Hispanic origin.

**Figure I.1** Ethnicity and national origin of the Asian American population, 2019.

*Source*: PEW Research Center. (2021, April 29). *Key facts about Asian Americans, a diverse and growing population*. https://www.pewresearch.org/fact-tank/2021/04/29/key-facts-about-asian-americans.

shows the ethnicity and national origin of the 2019 Asian American population.[10]

The remaining 15% of Asian Americans include individuals who identify as Pakistani, Cambodian, Hmong, Thai, Laotian, Taiwanese, Bangladeshi, Burmese, Indonesian, Nepalese, Sri Lankan, Malaysian, Mongolian, Bhutanese, and Okinawan.[11] It is estimated that there are almost 50 distinct Asian American ethnic groups speaking 30 different languages in the United States; therefore, the term *Asian American* refers to a highly diverse and distinct group of people with varying histories, cultures, views of mental illness, and beliefs about suicide.[12]

The Asian American population in the United States will continue to expand in the future. According to the Pew Research Center, the U.S. Asian population is projected to reach 46 million by 2060.[13] Similarly, the Asian American college student population will continue to grow in the years to come. For example, the number and proportion of Asian American college students grew exponentially during the past 30 years; in 2008, more than 1.3 million college students in the United States identified themselves as Asian American.[14] Moreover, the population of Asian American college students increased between 2000 and 2015, and it is projected that Asians will make up 14% of the total college population by 2024.[15]

Asian American college students reported higher levels of suicide ideation than European American college students.[16] For example, Asian American college students were 1.6 times more likely to have seriously considered attempting suicide than European American college students.[17] However, Asian Americans between the ages of 18 and 24 years have lower rates of suicide deaths than European Americans in the same age group.[18] For example, the suicide death rate for Asian American and Pacific Islander American individuals aged 18–24 years was 12.3%, whereas the suicide death rate for European American individuals in the same age group was 16.9%.[19] This age frame is generally the traditional age of most college students. Moreover, the Centers for Disease Control and Prevention categorizes Asian Americans and Pacific Island Americans into the same category; thus, the 12.3% figure will be lower for Asian Americans because it will also include the numbers for Pacific Islander Americans. The previous information indicates that Asian American college students are vulnerable to suicide ideation. However, they are also resilient to suicide deaths. This paradox of Asian American college students' suicide vulnerability and resiliency is worth examining in greater detail.

## The Paradox of Vulnerability and Resiliency

The suicide deaths of Asian American college students mostly from East Coast schools have received some public attention throughout the years. These case studies include Elizabeth Shin, a Korean American student at the Massachusetts Institute of Technology (MIT);[20] Luke Tang, a Chinese American student at Harvard University;[21] and Alexander Urtula, a Filipino American student at Boston College.[22] Further news reporting of Asian American college students on the East Coast who died by suicide provided disturbing information. First, more than half the suicide deaths between 1996 and 2006 at Cornell University were Asian or Asian American, whereas Asians only made up 14% of Cornell's student population.[23] Second, at MIT, 8 of the 19 suicide deaths (42%) in the past 15 years involved Asian American students, yet only 16% of the MIT students identified as Asian American.[24] Finally, between 2007 and 2017, there were 9 suicide deaths at Harvard University, including 6 students of Asian descent. However, Asian Americans only make up 20% of Harvard's undergraduate student body.[25] Asian American college student suicides made the news in other ways. The media coverage of the deadliest college shooting in the United States at Virginia Polytechnic Institute and State University, commonly referred to as Virginia Tech, in 2007 drew attention to the perpetrator, a Korean American college student who died by suicide after the mass shooting.[26] The news information was a bit silent on the West Coast colleges and universities. I found one piece of news that focused on a college in California. In this example, 3 Asian American students at the California Institute of Technology died by suicide within a 3-month period in 2009.[27]

## Suicide Vulnerability

The specific cases just mentioned highlight suicide vulnerability among Asian American college students. This is a cause for concern because there is a connection between suicide ideation and suicide death. For example, suicide ideation is a significant health concern because it can precede a suicide attempt.[28] Factors contributing to suicide ideation include hopelessness, loneliness, and helplessness. Furthermore, depressive symptoms predict suicidal thoughts.[29] In addition, depression is a serious illness that affects thoughts, feelings, and the ability to function in everyday life. It is one of the most common mental disorders in the United States, affecting all age groups. The fifth edition of the *Diagnostic and Statistical Manual of Mental Disorders,* text revision (DSM-5-TR), contains the most up-to-date criteria for identifying and understanding mental disorders. The DSM-5-TR has identified nine symptoms present in major depressive disorder (Box I.1).

---

### Box I.1 Major Depressive Disorder Diganostic Criteria

A. Five (or more) of the following symptoms have been present during the same 2-week period and represent a change from previous functioning; at least one of the symptoms is either (1) depressed mood or (2) loss of interest or pleasure.

**Note:** Do not include symptoms that are clearly attributable to another medical condition.

1. Depressed mood most of the day, nearly every day, as indicated by either subjective report (e.g., feels sad, empty, hopeless) or observation made by others (e.g., appears tearful). [**Note:** In children and adolescents, can be irritable mood.]
2. Markedly diminished interest or pleasure in all, or almost all, activities, most of the day, nearly every day (as indicated by either subjective account or observation).
3. Significant weight loss when not dieting or weight gain (e.g., a change of more than 5% of body weight in a month), or decrease or increase in appetite nearly every day. [**Note:** In children, consider failure to make expected weight gain.]
4. Insomnia or hypersomnia nearly every day.
5. Psychomotor agitation or retardation nearly every day (observable by others, not merely subjective feelings of restlessness or being slowed down).
6. Fatigue or loss of energy nearly every day.
7. Feelings of worthlessness or excessive or inappropriate guilt (which may be delusional) nearly every day (not merely self-reproach or guilt about being sick).
8. Diminished ability to think or concentrate, or indecisiveness, nearly every day (either by subjective account or as observed by others).

9. Recurrent thoughts of death (not just the fear of dying), recurrent suicidal ideation without a specific plan, or a suicide attempt or a specific plan for committing suicide.

B. The symptoms cause clinically significant distress or impairment in social, occupational, or other important areas of functioning.

C. The episode is not attributable to the physiological effects of a substance or another medical condition.
**Note:** Criteria A-C represent a major depressive episode.
**Note:** Responses to a significant loss (e.g., bereavement, financial ruin, losses from a natural disaster, a serious medical illness or disability) may include the feelings of intense sadness, rumination about the loss, insomnia, poor appetite, and weight loss noted in Criteria A, which may resemble a depressive episode. Although such symptoms may be understandable or considered appropriate to the loss, the present of a major depressive episode in addition to the normal response to a significant loss should be carefully considered. This decision inevitably requires the exercise of clinical judgment based on the individual's history and cultural norms for the expression of distress in the context of loss.

D. At least one major depressive episode is not better explained by schizoaffective disorder and is not superimposed on schizophrenia, schizophreniform disorder, delusional disorder, or other specified and unspecified schizophrenia spectrum and other psychotic disorders.

E. There has never been a manic episode or hypomanic episode.
**Note:** This exclusion does not apply if all of the manic-like or hypomanic-like episodes are substance-induced or are attributable to the physiological effects of another medical condition.

*Source:* Reprinted with permission from the *Diagnostic and Statistical Manual of Mental Disorders: Fifth Edition*, pp. 183–184 (Copyright © 2022). American Psychiatric Association. All Rights Reserved.

A diagnosis of major depressive disorder (or clinical depression) is made if an individual reports experiencing five or more of these symptoms in the same 2-week period. One indicator of major depressive disorder includes recurrent thoughts of death, recurrent suicidal ideation without a specific plan, or suicide attempt or a specific plan for dying by suicide.[30] Therefore, major depressive disorder is connected to suicide ideation.

The research on Asian American college students throughout the United States and suicide ideation is fairly consistent. As stated previously, Asian American college students reported higher levels of depression, anxiety, and suicide ideation than European American college students. There are several studies to explain why this may be the case. Asian American college students go through specific social experiences that may intensify their existing mental health challenges, including acculturative stress, intergenerational conflicts, and perceived racism.

First, acculturation is the process of acclimating to cultural and social changes; Acculturative stress reflects the emotional reaction to life events and activities associated with the process of acculturation. For students of color, acculturative stress comes with the college experience. One study found that college students of color experienced acculturative stress because they are forced to adapt to both the demanding academic environment and social pressures associated with college life as a student of color. For example, an acculturative stressor may include learning to become more proficient in the English language in order to do well in classes. Students may need to develop their speaking and writing skills to participate more fully in academic and social life in college. Students of color are also challenged with balancing competing cultural values that come from their family and campus environments. In this way, they are learning to find the balance between embracing their old life with their families and their new life with their campus community. Moreover, students of color need to manage the difficulties of experiencing discrimination from the dominant culture. These examples of acculturative stress are related to greater levels of social anxiety and suicidal symptoms among students of color, including Asian American college students who made up 32.5% of the sample population from this southwestern university. These students conveyed their sense of psychological struggle in college with these words: "I have more barriers to overcome than most people."[31]

Second, the continuing racism experienced by Asian American college students contributes to their psychological pain and suffering. Face-to-face interviews with Asian American college students were conducted at several colleges and universities throughout the United States to learn more about campus racism. Asian American college students discussed the various forms of campus discrimination, including their experiences in a racially hostile environment, the perpetual foreigner myth, and the model minority myth. For example, one student shared information about an Asian American friend who had human feces smeared on their dorm door. This targeted student was the only Asian American student on that floor. Although this incident did not happen to the person sharing the story, it had a chilling effect on them: "If it happens to another Asian American, I know that it can happen to me. . . . I've heard about so many other incidents like this. I know it can happen to me. That's how I'm personally affected by it."

In another incident, a different student shared a story about riding a bus when three European American college men came on the bus and shouted, "Hey. Is this even the American bus?" The student did not respond because "I didn't want to cause trouble or harm to myself." This student was very scared that the event could escalate into violence, but they were also very upset that they were singled out. Finally, another interviewee expressed frustration when current classmates complained that Asian American students have an academic advantage because they are more intelligent: "Whenever we get our midterms and I get a good grade, they're all like 'Dude. You're Asian. It's not fair.' I'm like 'What? I studied.'"[32] In these three interviews, Asian American college students explained that violence and racism were directed at them solely because they were perceived as Asian or Asian American.

Finally, there is evidence that Asian American college students experience psychological distress if they encounter intergenerational conflict, particularly with their parents. A sample of Asian American college students at a large West Coast public university indicated they seriously considered suicide when they experienced unfulfilled interpersonal expectations. For example, these students explained that their parents had extremely high expectations for them to achieve academic excellence. This placed a lot of pressure on the college students. When they were not able to succeed in the manner expected by their parents, they experienced severe psychological anguish and pain that included suicide ideation; these individuals seriously considered dying by suicide to end their suffering. This study concluded that parental pressures were the most common event preceding the students' development of suicide ideation. Furthermore, these parental conflicts associated the family unit as a risk factor for suicide-related outcomes among Asian American college students.[33]

These three studies together move forward the argument that Asian American students are deeply affected by negative social interactions within the family and campus environments during their time in college. In addition, these studies were published before the global pandemic. The more recent research conducted during the global pandemic demonstrated that there were exceptional social conditions that were experienced by the Asian American population that further aggravated their psychological challenges and difficulties.

The global pandemic negatively impacted just about everyone in the United States. For college students living in this time period, it was specifically disruptive to their classroom learning and college goals as they left campus to quarantine with family members at home. Adjusting to this new way of living and learning during the global pandemic further exacerbated mental health difficulties for college students. They were forced to transition to a virtual platform and engage in remote learning as they continued their studies. This practice led to prolonged periods of isolation and feelings of disconnection. Some students were returning to traumatic family situations in which they faced physical and psychological violence; these problematic family situations at home further intensified their existing mental health struggles.[34] Some students experienced financial insecurity, difficulty adjusting to online learning, or the loss of a loved one to COVID-19. For Asian Americans, there were additional—and more specific—problems and struggles.

Asian Americans were profoundly impacted during the global pandemic as they experienced continuing racism through the perpetual foreigner myth. This is a stereotype about Asian Americans regarding their perceived "otherness" that is not representative of American culture, values, and society; this opinion comes from European Americans who tend to equate "Americanness" with "Whiteness."[35] This othering of a specific racial group made it easier to blame Asian Americans for the spread of the coronavirus resulting in the global pandemic. Consequently, Asian Americans now experienced another dimension of racism: COVID-19 scapegoats.[36] Asian Americans were aggressively and irrationally targeted for the origins of the coronavirus, frequently resulting in violent attacks. As a result, the perpetual foreigner myth and scapegoating were connected forms of racism that Asian Americans experienced in this specific historical context.

Asians and Asian Americans were blamed for COVID-19, and this gave rise to more media coverage addressing anti-Asian hate. The nonprofit organization STOP APPI Hate was launched in March 2020 as a "response to the alarming escalation in xenophobia and bigotry resulting from the COVID-19 pandemic."[37] Furthermore, "this coalition tracks and responds to incidents of hate, violence, harassment, discrimination, shunning, and child bullying against Asian Americans and Pacific Islanders in the United States."[38] This organization received 9,081 incident reports between March 2020 and August 2021 regarding verbal harassment, shunning, and physical assaults.[39] In 2021, the Pew Research Center found that 8 in 10 Asian Americans stated that violence against them in the United States is increasing; nearly half experienced an incident connected to their racial or ethnic background since the beginning of the pandemic. Some of these confrontations included being subjected to racial slurs or jokes, blamed for the coronavirus outbreak, and told that they should go back to their home country.[40] These acts of aggression and hate continued to take a psychological toll on Asians and Asian Americans. On the college level, the pandemic brought to light familiar conversations about mental health struggles among students and their access to mental health resources.

Asian American college students are less likely to receive professional mental health support. One study collected information on mental health seeking before the global pandemic among Asian American and European American students from 70 colleges and universities in the United States. Approximately 39% of Asian Americans and 49% of European Americans sought professional psychological help for suicide ideation. In addition, Asian American and European American college students disclosed their suicide ideation to at least one person for the purpose of seeking social support; however, only 19% of Asian Americans, in contrast to 31% of European Americans, were advised by at least one person to seek professional support for their suicide ideation.[41] Therefore, fewer Asian American college students were encouraged by their loved ones to consider the possibility of seeking professional psychological resources and support.

There are other specific reasons Asian American college students are less likely to pursue professional psychological services. For example, Asian American college students reported greater general barriers to help-seeking, higher concerns with the loss of face, and higher family stigma toward mental health than European American college students.[42] Asian American college students also did not pursue professional mental health support because they did not want to be perceived as a burden to counselors and therapists. This sense of perceived burdensomeness was connected to the viewpoint that receiving support from mental health professionals would bring shame to one's family.[43] Although Asian American college students are less likely to receive mental health treatment than the general college population, they also have lower suicide death rates than the general college population.

*Suicide Resiliency*

The data consistently show lower rates of suicide deaths among the Asian American population aged 18–24 years, the general age of college students.[44] The 2019 population-based data indicate that Asian and Pacific Islander Americans aged 18–24 years have a lower rate of suicide deaths than most other racial groups. The suicide death rate per 100,000 individuals by racial classification was 16.9% White, 12.81% Black, 24.46% American Indian, and 12.37% Asian and Pacific Islander. Table I.1 shows the suicide death rate by race.

It is useful to note that this collected information does not disaggregate all racial data. For example, Asians and Pacific Islanders are pooled into one racial category. By contrast, the U.S. Census Bureau classifies Asian Americans as those with origins in the East, Southeast Asia, or the Indian Subcontinent; Native Hawaiians and Other Pacific Islanders are classified as those within the U.S. jurisdictions of Melanesia, Micronesia, and Polynesia.[45] These specific numbers do not tell the full story of suicide ideation and suicide deaths among Asian American college students. There are many Asian American college students who experience suicidal ideation, tendencies, and behaviors who do not die by suicide.

# Risk Factors and Vulnerability

One of the things I wanted to understand was the specific vulnerabilities experienced by the Asian American population. I wanted to learn more about the risk factors for suicide ideation that were specific or common to the Asian American college

**Table I.1** Suicide Death Rate by Race, 2019

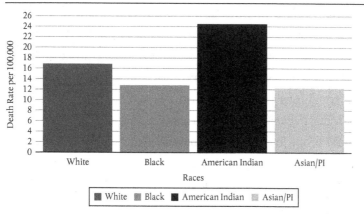

Applied Filters:
Suicide All Injury Deaths
State: All States
Race: All Races
Ethnicity: All Ethnicities
Sec: All Sexes
Year Range: Year Range: 2019–2019
Age Range: Age Range: 18–24

*Source*: Centers for Disease Control and Prevention–WISQARS. (n.d.). *Causes of injury-related death.* https://wisqars.cdc.gov/data/explore-data/explore/selected-years?ex=eyJoYmkiOlsiMCJdLCJpbnRlbnRzIjpbIjAiXSwibWVjaHMiOlsiMjA4M TAiXSwic3RhdGUiOlsiMDEiLCIwMiIsIjAoIiwiMDUiLCIwNiIsIjA4IiwiMDkiLCIx MCIsIjExIiwiMTIiLCIxMyIsIjE1IiwiMTYiLCINyIsIjE4IiwiMTkiLCIyMCIsIjIxIiwiM jIiLCIyMyIsIjIoIiwiMjUiLCIyNiIsIjI3IiwiMjgiLCIyOSIsIjMwIiwiMzEiLCIzMiIsIjMz IiwiMzQiLCIzNSIsIjM2IiwiMzciLCIzOCIsIjM5IiwiNDAiLCIoMSIsIjQyIiwiNDQiL CIoNSIsIjQ2IiwiNDciLCIoOCIsIjQ5IiwiNTAiLCI1MSIsIjUzIiwiNTQiLCI1NSIsIjU 2IlosInJhY2UiOlsiMSIsIjIiLCIzIiwiNCJdLCJldGGhuaWNoeSI6WyIxIiwiMiIsIjMiXS wic2V4IjpbIjEiLCIyIlosImFnZUdyb3Vwco1pbiI6WyIwMCowNCJdLCJhZ2VHcm 91cHNNYXgiOlsiMTk5IlosImN1c3RvbUFnZXNNaW4iOlsiMTgiXSwiY3VzdG9tQ Wdlco1heCI6WyIyNCJdLCJmcm9tWWVhci6WyIyMDE5IlosInRvWWVhci6Wy IyMDE5IlosInlwbGxBZ2VzIjpbIjYillosIm1ldHJvIjpbIjEiLCIyIlosImFnZWJucdHRuI joiY3VzdG9tIiwiZ3JvdXBieTEiOiJOT05FIno%3D.

population. What accounted for their high degrees of suicide ideation? What were the external and social factors that contributed to their psychological distress? How did they experience the world differently from other college students? The sociologist Emile Durkheim demonstrated that individual struggles are rooted in social conditions and that the field of sociology can scientifically study social behavior. Durkheim analyzed suicide data in different areas of Europe in the 19th century and identified the lack of social integration as a contributing factor to suicide deaths. As a result, he explained that the cause of suicide death was an individual's lack of social connectedness in society.

Durkheim used the term *egoistic suicide* to describe the prolonged negative experience of not belonging in a community. An isolated individual who is not socially participating with other human beings will develop feelings of meaninglessness, apathy, and unhappiness. Durkheim called such social detachment "excessive individuation." These individuals are not sufficiently bound to social groups and are left with little social support or guidance. He indicated that this type of suicide occurred among unmarried people, especially unmarried men, whom he found had less to bind and connect them to stable social norms and goals. Therefore, an individual's low degree of social integration in a community contributed to suicidal behaviors and suicide deaths.[46] This lack of social bonding and cohesion is further explained by psychologist Thomas Joiner.

Joiner further developed Durkheim's concept of social integration by identifying thwarted belongingness and perceived burdensomeness as contributing factors to suicide ideation.[47] Thwarted belongingness has been described as an individual's perception that they are isolated from others and do not form a vital part of a valued social group; therefore, an individual's need to belong is unfulfilled because they do not experience positive interactions with a certain group of individuals in a caring, sustained, and nurturing environment.[48] The main premise of thwarted belongingness is indicated with the statement, "I am alone."[49] Thwarted belongingness calls attention to loneliness, including living alone and having few social supports. In addition, reciprocal care is absent, meaning that an individual lacks a social support system and is not considered a part of another's social support system.[50] Accordingly, the main consideration for thwarted belongingness is social isolation.

The feelings of thwarted belongingness are connected to racial oppression and marginalization. Political scientist Iris Young explained that the marginalization of nondominant racial groups expels them from full participation in social life. Racial discrimination is an example of marginalization: "Increasingly in the United States racial oppression occurs in the form of marginalization rather than exploitation. Marginalization is perhaps the most dangerous form of oppression."[51] For example, Asian Americans continue to negotiate direct and indirect forms of racial discrimination from childhood through adulthood in the United States. One study established that Asian American males endured chronic racial discrimination that resulted in repeated acts of racial trauma.[52] Consequently, constant exposure to racial discrimination is associated with higher rates of mental and physical health problems.[53] In addition, Asian Americans have experienced specific acts of racism within the broader context of the United States. For example, there was a rise in anti-Asian sentiment during the global pandemic, including negative tweets on Twitter,[54] discriminatory rhetoric in American political speeches,[55] and a surge in hate crimes targeting Asian Americans.[56]

Joiner also recognizes that thwarted belongingness is connected to perceived burdensomeness. Perceived burdensomeness refers to the perception that one is a burden to family members, friends, or society; the individual believes that personal flaws become a social liability.[57] The main premise of perceived burdensomeness is indicated with the statement, "I am a burden."[58] The feelings of perceived burdensomeness include two important concepts: liability and self-hate. Liability involves the feeling that one is expendable and unessential because one is a burden to others; it is the conviction that one's death is worth more than one's life to others. Furthermore, the experiences of self-hate involve feelings of low self-esteem, anxiety, and deep shame.[59] The feelings of perceived burdensomeness are a significant risk factor for Asian Americans. The perception that one is a burden to one's family unit or extended kinship is particularly devastating for communities that value family cohesion and interconnection.[60] The solidarity and harmony in a household may be compromised when an individual believes they are not living up to the expectations and obligations of the family unit. For example, one study explained that Asian American students suffered with tremendous pressure from their parents to achieve academic excellence; consequently, these students experienced criticism, guilt, or shame when they underperformed academically and disappointed their parents.[61]

Asian American students experience feelings of perceived burdensomeness when they live with mental illness. In some cultures, depression and other forms of mental illnesses are viewed as a sign of personal weakness and bring shame to the family.[62] In some Asian American families, it was not proper to share personal feelings, struggles, or problems. One study specified that Asian Americans have difficulty discussing personal problems with family members because they are socialized to not openly express emotions; rather, they are encouraged to practice shyness, restraint, and subordination. Because they are discouraged from expressing their feelings and emotions, individuals believe they are a liability to their family due to their limitations, shortcomings, and weaknesses.[63] In turn, sensing a weak connection to the family may bring about feelings of distress and insecurity as well as increase the vulnerability to depression.[64] Together, the theoretical contributions from Durkheim, Joiner, and Young helped me develop a framework to organize the concepts of risk and vulnerability to further explore suicide ideation among Asian American college students.

## Protective Factors and Resiliency

The other thing I wanted to understand about the Asian American population was how they managed their suicide ideation. I wanted to learn more about the protective factors against suicide death that were specific or common to the Asian American college population. What accounted for their low rates of suicide deaths? What were the external and social factors that contributed to their psychological resiliency? How did they experience the world differently from other college students? The theoretical lens of resiliency helped me frame an understanding of the protective factors that may contribute to the prevention of suicide deaths. Resiliency theories draw from multiple disciplines and address a range of processes for developing human strength and vitality. For the purpose of this book, *resiliency* is defined in the broadest sense to include determination, resolve, and persistence. In this way, human resiliency is the ability to adapt successfully in the face of stress and adversity.[65] In addition, resiliency theories have addressed suicide ideation: "Resilience factors are psychological attributes, processes, or abilities that attenuate the negative impact of risk factors, thereby diminishing the probability of suicidal outcomes in situations of adversity"[66] Therefore, resiliency theories focus on a person's ability to function competently by reducing the risk factors to manage their mental health challenges.

The theoretical lens of resiliency examines individuals, groups, and communities from a strength-based perspective rather than from a deficit-based perspective. Whereas a deficit-based perspective focuses on the problem of an individual, a strength-based perspective focuses on the attributes of an individual as part of the healing process.[67] I am writing this book from a strength-based perspective. When I was reviewing the suicide literature on Asian Americans, I did not find many articles focusing on the management of their suicide ideation. Although I learned the many causes and factors that contributed to their psychological distress, I did not find out how they used their personal abilities and other resources to learn how to live with mental health challenges. This seemed to me a very important component of a suicidal person's story. This was the story I wanted to hear, and it was the story I wanted to tell. For these reasons, it was my goal to write this book from the perspectives of hope, possibility, and courage. In doing so, I was inspired by the scholars before me. For example, it has been noted that earlier research on child and adolescent development focused primarily on negative elements such as identifying risk factors in the formative years. However, Zimmerman took a strength-based approach to understanding child and adolescent health by focusing on the positive factors in a young person's life, including self-efficacy and self-esteem.[68] Furthermore, this study indicated that young people also found support through youth programs, as well as from their parents and mentors. Other works have also used a strength-based approach to emphasize the resiliency of young people, including suicidal homeless youth[69] and suicidal middle school students.[70]

For the purpose of this book, the three most relevant elements of resiliency are coping strategies, support systems, and life skills. First, coping strategies are processes that help develop individual resiliency during times of psychological distress. Coping focuses on "one's cognitive and behavioral efforts to manage specific external and/or internal demands that are appraised as taxing or exceeding the resources of the person."[71] The path to developing psychological resilience is an active and mindful process that continues over a period of time. It is an evolving journey in which the psychologically distressed person cultivates the strength, resolve, and endurance to manage the challenges and struggles in daily life. Specifically, the process of using psychological and behavioral techniques to manage, reduce, and overcome stress has been linked to resilience.[72] A common coping strategy is self-reliance. Self-reliance holds the perspective that even during an emotional or psychological crisis, an individual must be strong, determined, and self-directed above and beyond what has already been endured.[73] One research study explained that individual coping strategies in the moment focused on quiet activities such as mediating and journal writing. Other individual coping strategies in the moment included using physical objects to release their frustrations, including slamming doors, flipping over furniture, or screaming into pillows. All of these examples used self-reliance as a coping strategy to release pain and stress.[74]

Second, social support is considered a protective factor against suicidal behavior and suicide deaths. The presence of social support and the behavior of seeking social support have been associated with psychological hardiness and flourishing in the face of major adverse life events.[75] Furthermore, there is evidence that social support might protect individuals from suicidal tendencies by increasing feelings of belongingness, which are negatively associated with suicide risk.[76] For example, researchers surveyed 379 college students, 18% of whom were Asian American, and found that social support from family, friends, and significant others substantially reduced the feelings of suicide ideation.[77] Having a strong support system was particularly important during the early phases of the global pandemic. In this time period, college students experienced profound social isolation, loneliness, and disconnection. As they were leaving their college campuses for home, they were also reminded to monitor their well-being and engage in meaningful human interaction. College students were encouraged to use technology to their advantage by spending a few minutes talking with people they care about on a regular basis. Even a few minutes in conversation with a loved one would be fulfilling and would provide some moments of joy and happiness.[78]

Finally, life skills are essential to human development and survival. Life skills include basic activities such as managing nutrition, sleep, money, possessions, and time. These are essential proficiencies and abilities that individuals learn over the course of their lives. To live a healthy and substantial life, individuals are encouraged to take more responsibility for self-care and self-management as they evolve and develop in the adulthood years.[79] Self-care is a productive life skill that involves cultivating intentional healthy habits and practices each day. The research on college students and health indicated that making time for personal wellness and lifestyle habits increased one's commitment to self-care. Self-care includes being mindful and aware of one's human needs. For example, college students were encouraged to monitor their daily physical activities and to examine their eating habits as practices of mindfulness.[80] Collective mindfulness and compassion include the awareness of the self and the awareness of others; it embraces an attitude of openness, curiosity, and trust through the care for self and others. In other words, enhanced mindfulness is a practice that increased self-compassion and well-being.[81]

The contributions from Durkheim, Joiner, and Young along with the theoretical lens of resiliency developed the conceptual framework for this book. The concepts of social integration, thwarted belongingness, and perceived burdensomeness provide the framework to examine the risk factors to suicide ideation, suicidal behaviors, and suicide deaths. These risk factors explain the suicide vulnerability of Asian American college students. The theoretical lens of resiliency focused on the protective factors of suicide ideation and deaths by emphasizing coping strategies, support systems, and life skills. These protective factors explain the suicide resiliency of Asian American college students. Figure I.2 shows the conceptual framework for examining Asian American college students' experiences with suicide vulnerability and resiliency.

Using this conceptual framework, my study explored the following research questions:

1. What is the experience of suicide ideation among Asian American college students?
2. How do Asian American college students who experience suicide ideation develop suicide resiliency by using coping strategies, support systems, and life skills to work through suicidal tendencies during their time in college?

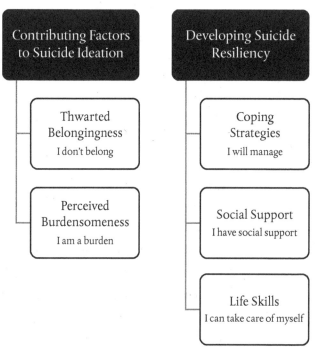

**Figure I.2** Conceptual framework for examining Asian American college students' experiences with suicide ideation and resiliency.

I used narrative research to understand the experiences of suicide vulnerability and suicide resiliency among Asian American college students. Specifically, I focused on the risk factors to explain suicide vulnerability and the protective factors to explain suicide resiliency. The first research question addressed the risk factors to describe their vulnerability to suicide ideation. The second research question addressed the protective factors to describe their resiliency to suicide deaths. In order to explore these factors, I needed to find and recruit Asian American college students who were willing to share their experiences of psychological pain and endurance.

INTRODUCTION

# A Collection of Human Stories

There were two requirements to participate in my study. First, college students needed to identify as Asian American. Second, these college students expressed suicide ideation at some point in their lives. Narrative research involves detailed and thorough individual interviews. The core of comprehensive interviews is to understand the lived experiences of individuals and the meaning they make of those experiences.[82] The specific strategy of narrative research is to discover the meaning, context, and process of lived human experiences.[83] Through this practice, the participants and I were involved in a sustained and intensive process through storytelling.[84] In addition, this storytelling process generated a relationship between the person who told the story and me, the person who listened to the story. Therefore, narrative research is the process of trying to make sense of people's stories and recognizing that each human being has a story worth sharing.[85]

The process of storytelling and listening comes from a strong tradition among communities of color. It is the recognition that each person's story is important and powerful. Each piece of information that gets shared contributes to a collective story in which every person who shares that experience, culture, or understanding has a place of connectedness and belongingness. Furthermore, the theme of a story tells us something about that person's culture and history. Different narratives are shared for different reasons. For example, storytelling includes stories of survival.[86] Sharing stories about our survival is a way of demonstrating active resistance toward the obstacles that get in the way of our survival. Telling our stories of struggle is a way to celebrate our survival; it is a way of honoring our individual journey of perseverance in the face of profound adversity. Celebrating our survival is a deeply human experience: "Celebrating is a natural outcome of spiritual sharing and it too can take a diversity of forms. It is an individual and communal process that celebrates the mystery of life and the journey that each of us takes."[87]

The way to honor our survival is through the engagement of storytelling. Letting the storyteller share their experiences means the person listening to the words must be respectful when asking questions. There are some questions that are not culturally appropriate to ask of individuals. There may also be some questions to which the answers are too painful for the storyteller to share. Therefore, it is important to consider what to refuse in the story-sharing process.

The progression of sharing personal accounts may be a reflective and traumatic experience. As a researcher, I was reminded to practice compassion because the manner of engaging in serious conversations may involve pain and humiliation for the individuals telling their stories. Moreover, individuals sharing their personal suffering and challenges are entrusting their memories to me as I re-story their life experiences.[88] Restorying is a method of analyzing the participants' stories by reorganizing the statements, descriptions, and explanations into some general type of framework.[89] This framework will use categories to organize the major themes of the research findings. Moreover, the person listening to the story has the opportunity to refuse to ask certain questions as well as refuse to include certain sensitive information when writing the final report. The practice of refusing is a more compassionate method to collecting information from the storytellers, the research participants.[90] It honors the dignity of each person and respects that not all stories are told for mass public consumption. In communities in which certain stories are not shared with people outside those communities, it is a mindful practice to respect that not all information will be shared to a broader audience.

This is the path I have taken to ensure the confidentiality of each participant. Some profile information have been removed so that participants will not be identified in this book. Thus, I have provided a limited sketch of each college student. Similarly, I designated a pseudonym for each person and have addressed them with the inclusive pronoun "they." Finally, it was my practice to be respectful of all participants by asking only the questions that were truly needed to address the research questions.[91]

All 12 participants self-identified as Asian American college students between the ages of 18 and 23 years who have expressed experiences with depression and/or suicide ideation. Table I.2 shows their current age and self-identified ethnicities.

This book consists of three chapters. Chapter 1 highlights suicide vulnerability. It offers a discussion on the risk factors of suicide ideation. In this chapter, I emphasize the six risk factors of psychological distress and suicide ideation: a history of mental health challenges, the impact of a bad day, intergenerational trauma, thwarted belongingness, and perceived burdensomeness. Chapter 2 focuses on suicide resiliency. It examines the protective factors of suicide deaths. In this chapter, I concentrate on the six protective factors that develop a person's suicide resiliency: living

Table I.2  Self-Identified Ethnicity and Age of Interview Participants

| Participant | Self-Identified Ethnicity | Age (Years) |
|---|---|---|
| Alex | Vietnamese | 21 |
| Cameron | Japanese | 20 |
| Dana | Chinese | 19 |
| Evelyn | Half Korean, the other half is a mixture of South Asian and White | 20 |
| Hayden | Filipino | 20 |
| Jamie | Chinese | 21 |
| Kelly | Filipino | 23 |
| Morgan | A mix of Chinese and White | 20 |
| Quinn | Korean | 18 |
| Robin | Chinese Vietnamese | 22 |
| Shannon | Filipino | 23 |
| Taylor | Laotian Vietnamese | 21 |

through the global pandemic, coping strategies and self-reliance, support systems and human attachment, life skills and self-care, the impact of a good day, and reasons for living. Finally, Chapter 3 addresses the paradox of suicide vulnerability and resiliency. In this chapter, I summarize my research findings and offer both practice and research recommendations.

# CHAPTER 1

# THE RISK FACTORS FOR SUICIDE IDEATION

The American Association of Suicidology published a handbook for people who have lost a loved one to suicide. This 36-page handbook offers a position called the accumulation of pain to explain suicidal emotions:

> Suicidal depression is pain that seems to "accumulate" from many experiences. While most people find ways to cope with life's common difficulties, the suicidal person—while seeming to move past each setback, loss, and misfortune—continues to carry pain from each trauma with them throughout their lives. With each new hurt both great and small, a little more pain is added to this tragic cargo until it becomes unbearable.[1]

One way to help organize this way of thinking is to consider that the outcome of suicide is not to end life but, rather, to end deep suffering. Accumulated pain may occur over the course of a person's life. Continued disappointments and challenges add up to diminish a person's confidence and happiness; over time, the individual feels compromised and destroyed from all the failures. Prolonged disappointments experienced over and over again shatter us. When we are broken, we do not feel whole. These

*Stories of Survival.* Amy Wong, Oxford University Press. © Oxford University Press 2023.
DOI: 10.1093/oso/9780197662397.003.0002

ongoing challenges seem never to end, and they make it even more difficult for individuals with prolonged mental health struggles.

## History of Mental Health Challenges

Participants who experienced suicide ideation while in college had a history of depression and hopelessness in middle school and high school. They explained that these persisting suicidal tendencies included negative thoughts, invalidating feelings, and destructive behaviors. Most individuals recalled specific periods in their life when suicide ideation was more evident and pronounced. Revisiting their middle school and high school memories several years later, they were able to remember vivid details about their experiences with psychological distress. For many, it was a confusing, uncertain, and lonely period. Hayden, who aspires to become an occupational therapist, recalled moving every few years while living in Japan and the United States because their father was in the military. As they were going through puberty in middle school, they experienced confusion about who they were but did not have many friends to share these troubling feelings. They internalized their disturbing feelings and experienced suicide ideation. At the same time, their parents' high academic expectations generated profound psychological distress and greatly contributed to their suicidal thoughts in the middle school years:

> Looking back, I don't know why it was like that because it's just middle school, and colleges don't look at middle school, but that's where it started getting tough, and I felt as a middle schooler there was just too much pressure on me. That's when I started thinking, "Oh, my God, I just can't do this." I can't go to them. I can't go to

anyone else because I'm so used to moving, and I'm so used to just being friendly and making friends and then forgetting about them because I'm only here for a few years or they're only here for a few years. I don't have anyone else to talk to. I can't go to my parents. My sister is still a kid, so she can't quite relate to me, at least in my opinion. I just felt really lonely, and I just wanted to . . . I just had the idea of suicide.

Several students did not understand what they were going through in the middle school and high school years; they described how they did not have the language to express their emotional and psychological suffering. They only knew that they were in pain; however, they did not know how to address the pain. In addition, these young adults believed their tormenting ordeal was a common teenage experience for other middle schoolers and high schoolers. They did not believe that what they were going through was special or unique because they speculated that they might grow out of these feelings as they got older. However, they found that these negative feelings did not go away as they got older. In time, they developed a better understanding of their younger life as they learned the language for their feelings and emotions. For example, Jamie reflected on their earlier school experiences and discussed how they did not identify as a depressed or suicidal person in middle school. They only knew that, sometimes, they wanted to die:

> When I was in middle school, I didn't know what it was. I didn't identify it within myself that I was depressed or suicidal. I just knew that, sometimes, I was just thinking about killing myself or, sometimes, I just felt like, you know, I don't want to be here. I don't need to be here. What am I doing here? What am I contributing to anything in this world? And I didn't know it at the time that I was

feeling those things as a suicidal person. I just thought that they were regular thoughts that came to me.

Living with depressive emotions in their earlier years was a distressing existence for college students. They expressed feelings of loneliness because they were not able to talk with family members or close friends about their deep-rooted emotional and mental pain. This sense of isolation further contributed to their mental anguish, and many individuals suffered in silence by themselves. Students recalled the need to release some of this psychological suffering by talking to a human being. Jamie remembered this lonely and traumatic time: "I have gotten to very, very low points in my life where I needed to call the suicide hotline because I really had no one else to talk to." The need for a human connection was deeply desired by the participants. Their psychological pain was compounded when they did not have people in their daily lives. The feelings of loneliness and the lack of human connection made their suffering more devastating. Dana experienced profound feelings of isolation as their friends left their life, one by one:

> The feelings of hopelessness tend to come around when I'm feeling lonely. I know that I have friends out there, but it doesn't always feel like I have people. At the beginning of my senior year of high school, I felt like I lost a lot of friends just from circumstantial stuff. One of them got a boyfriend, and she started hanging out with him all the time. Another one of my close friends, she got into a ballet program as a trainee, and I was very proud, but she had to drop out to finish high school online. She was one of my closest friends, and then she left. Another one of my close friends, we had a bit of a falling out. We're okay now. It was just a rough period when I felt there were few people in my corner.

Without someone to talk with, several of the participants tried to work through their mental disturbances by themselves. They found ways to diminish the emotional suffering by seeking comfort and pleasure in specific activities. Some found comfort in unhealthy habits such as overindulging in food; however, this addictive practice ultimately made them feel ashamed about their bodies. One student talked about food as a source of pleasure and pain: "Sometimes I would eat a lot, and I would binge. At first, it gave me comfort; however, after that, it just kind of made me feel worse because it made me feel bad about my body." Binge eating is an addictive disorder that is difficult to control. Addictive disorders develop over time, and individuals may find pleasure and comfort in these activities because they alleviate short-term suffering.[2] Over time, these addictions are unhealthy for the body and mind. Eating disorders further contribute to a person's mental and physical struggle, and it becomes a battle that one has with themselves as they try to battle the addiction. Addictive disorders also complicate relationships with other people and lead to deteriorating social relationships. For example, Alex developed an eating disorder in high school, and this further caused difficulties in the relationship with their parents while they were making their college decision:

I developed an eating disorder, and that caused a lot of internal trauma. My family made me feel bad. I was just fighting it mentally, and that caused me to have a lot of anxiety and depression. I was just in a really dark place. My parents were kind of leaning towards not letting me go to college and making me take a gap year. I feel that coming from another state and not knowing anyone and starting new made it especially difficult for me to kind of adapt. I think that kind of made my depression a lot worse freshman year.

I was kind of just trying to go day by day, trying to focus on school, to kind of ignore my other issues. I felt really hopeless and alone.

The feelings of hopelessness and loneliness in high school continued into the college years. Although some individuals explained that suicide ideation was more intense in high school than in college, the overall transition to college campus life was demanding and it made it more difficult to manage their suicidal tendencies. For Kelly, suicidal thoughts were more pronounced in high school, but they were more problematic in the college years. When asked when they experienced suicide ideation, they stated, "I felt more of it in high school, but it definitely carried over into college in ways that I didn't expect. And it happened a lot of times when I did not need it." Although it is never a convenient time to experience suicide ideation, students were quick to point out that the college schedule and activities were more demanding and challenging; therefore, the busy schedule made it more difficult to address their suicidal tendencies.

For some students, suicidal thoughts were more fleeting, and for others, they were more prolonged. Students who experienced more short-term suicide ideation were able to identify a specific experience that influenced their suicidal thoughts. For Morgan, the suicidal thoughts were short-lived and usually occurred after an argument with their parents: "You just get into one of those huge fights, and it's just like I want to make it all go away, but then 5 minutes later, it's gone." For others, the suicidal thoughts were more pronounced and sustained. Students who experienced more long-term suicide ideation did not identify a particular experience that made them feel suicidal; rather, they talked about more general feelings of pain, anguish, and torment. Cameron remembered feeling great sadness for no particular reason at age 10 years and tying a cord around their neck to try to end the pain. They elaborated on the challenges of growing up with severe anxiety and living in a household that did not understand the concept of mental illness. Cameron spent about half of their life struggling with hopelessness, depression, and suicide ideation. Each day for about a year, they imagined they could end their deep suffering in one specific way:

> I do remember a period of time where I just genuinely did not want to live at the age of 17. I woke up every day thinking that I wanted to be hit by a car. I would walk to school, and I always imagined every morning that if I just make one step left, I can end it all right now. It was like that every single day for about a year. And mixed with my natural tendencies to just go lower and lower, mentally, it kind of convoluted itself into this big hole of I don't want to do this anymore.

Similarly, other students expressed feelings of continued profound pain. Evelyn found the mental health challenges that started in high school too great to handle alone in college. They have experienced depression, anxiety, and panic disorders. Evelyn discussed their mental health diagnosis and the need for mental health support in the high school years. The transition from high school to college was made more difficult because of ongoing mental health struggles that continued as they longed for the home environment that they left behind. For Evelyn, it was not enough to have the support of family members and friends; they needed the help of mental health professionals. After their earlier suicide attempt, they found the need for a team of mental health care providers during the college years:

I've actually been diagnosed with major depressive disorder, and on top of that generalized anxiety disorder and panic disorder. So, I have experience with depression since high school. I went into college not resolving the issues I already had, so it kind of made it worse. I was feeling homesick. I was missing my home life. I felt very isolated in the dorm. I wasn't getting help before the attempt because I stopped seeing my therapist in high school, and I went into college not having a therapist. I didn't want any help. I didn't want to do anything. I just wanted to sit there and do nothing, but I was hospitalized. So, I kind of was forced to get help, but I definitely needed the help. So, I have a team for my mental health now.

The psychological pain these students experienced in middle school and high school did not go away in college; rather, these negative thoughts and feelings persisted in college as they left the safety of their family home life to begin a new life in a different environment. In this new learning space, they experienced being homesick, a more academically challenging environment, and new cultural and social adjustments. Looking back on some of their early college days, participants talked about happy and sad moments. They discussed their good and bad days. These bad days further contributed to their overall mental health struggles and added to their accumulation of suffering.

## "Today Is a Bad Day"

The accumulation of rough days added to the overall stress of a person's life. The next day can be seen as a reset for challenges or troubles in a day, but over time, the accumulated struggles, disappointments, and pain take a toll on a person's mental health. In my interviews, participants talked about these accumulated bad days that contributed to an overall imbalance to feeling good. These setbacks chipped away at their confidence or happiness. Although many could regroup in the days to follow, a particularly bad day was more challenging to recover from. These difficult days were paralyzing and overwhelming particularly when a person had a history of mental health challenges.

All interview participants shared the qualities and elements that made for a bad day. They highlighted that sometimes they felt so overwhelmed and exhausted that they were not motivated to do anything at all. Quinn shared these feelings:

> If I have too much on my plate, instead of trying to get it done, I end up not doing any of it because it seems like so much at once. I'm too overwhelmed to do any of my work.

The experiences of feeling overburdened were summarized by Evelyn: "I don't have the motivation to do anything." Specifically, interviewees expressed the feelings of being overwhelmed with academic pressures, including earning poor grades, comparing themselves to other students, and not being able to get tasks done. These students stated that a bad day included not feeling in control of the day's activities. Alex explained the importance of a structured day:

> A bad day for me is a day where I'm disorganized, and things don't go as planned. I'm a very structured person and, a lot of times, if things don't go as planned or expected for me, it kind of really messes with my mood for the rest of the day. I'm really hard on myself. I wake up, and I forget about some assignment or the thing with my car, something like when things are not in my control that happened to me. Somehow, I'm late for class or I'm getting coffee,

and the person's taking forever. That kind of thing will kind of make my day worse.

Students expressed particular challenges with learning from remote spaces during the pandemic. They started the spring semester on campus but were moved to remote learning a few weeks into the new term. In addition to navigating a new world with confusing information, the abrupt move back home was disruptive for their studies. Once they returned home, they were isolated from their friends and had to use learning management systems to receive their lessons. Some students lost contact with their professors as faculty were also learning how to move their course content to an online platform. In general, students felt very alone as they spent hours in their rooms using the computer screens as their main source for learning. They were worn out with the many hours spent in distance learning and "being on Zoom for about 9 hours, 10 hours" each day. Dana discussed the academic challenges before and during the pandemic that contributed to their overall mood for the day:

> If I wake up late for class and arrived late because I like to be a punctual person. If I get a bad grade back, that usually kind of dampens the mood of the day. Sometimes, especially now, when I feel isolated because there're some days where I barely leave my room. I'm either in lectures or I'm doing homework, that kind of stuff. Then I realize it's like 9 p.m., and I haven't even left my apartment.

The interview participants did not look forward to the academic ritual of exam days. They did not enjoy the stress of studying for exams, and they did not like taking exams. These negative feelings would emerge in the days and weeks leading up to the exam period, which made them anxious and nervous. They also felt agitated and scared on the day of the exam as well as while taking the exam. In particular, they found the period of finals week stressful because of the prolonged time of taking one exam after another. Cameron did not look forward to "every day of finals week." Taylor highlighted the stress that comes with exam days:

> I don't think any of my classes have ever given me assurance if I've done well on an exam after coming out of it. Most of the time, I do okay, but just the experience of taking an exam makes me really uncomfortable. I really love learning and have a passion for learning but having to perform on an exam day really scares me.

Some students talked about having a negative classroom experience as contributing to a bad day. One example of a negative classroom experience was not having friends in the classroom and feeling alone. They did not enjoy sitting by themselves, and they found that it was not always easy to make friends in the classroom even though they had regular contact with their classmates. Students expressed a sense that classmates either started out as a friend group or that other classmates had an easier time making friends than they did. The overall feeling was that they were not welcomed in these classroom spaces, and they felt challenged to make new friends. Robin discussed not feeling welcomed in the classroom space and feeling trepidation about reaching out to other classmates:

> It's a bad day when I go to the class, and I didn't find anyone that I know in there. So, I'm thinking who I will talk to. The professor may require that we find a person or a student in the room, and then we have to discuss a topic. Most people like taking the class together with their friends, so they already have a group. I have to

work and get out of my comfort zone to ask people, "Hey, can I be in your group? Do you have a group?" That's maybe a bad day for me because I'm not an outside person. I am very much an inside person.

These feelings of being invisible in the classroom took a toll on their self-esteem. Students believed they had to make the effort to be friendly because they did not feel welcomed among other college students in the classroom. Similarly, Shannon talked about feeling invisible at their place of work:

> A bad day is when I don't feel welcomed at work, or I don't feel I'm basically wanted. I feel like I'm really good at reading the energy in the room, and from personal experience, there have been some times in my former job I felt like I walked into a space where I either felt invisible or not needed. Those are the days that were super bad.

Classroom challenges, academic difficulties, and workplace isolation contributed to a bad day for college students. These feelings of not feeling welcomed or not feeling a sense of belonging on a daily or weekly basis impacted their sense of well-being. They lived with these challenges on a daily and weekly basis with no end in sight. These days became repetitive. They also discussed the cycle of never-ending work; one bad day could be followed by another bad day. Jamie shared this pattern of a bad day that never seemed to end:

> A bad day for me would be sleeping at 5 a.m. and then waking up a couple hours later. I'm starting the day tired and then rushing to class without my coffee, then falling asleep in class. As well as missing an assignment and forgetting things that I need from home, such as pencils or my laptop. And then it's probably raining. Those are the worst days because then you're unprepared and just

not having the motivation to do any of the things that made me feel better, like not working out and just watching TV, probably just sitting around my room, feeling unproductive. And then stressing out about being unproductive, which makes me feel worse, and then staying up all night again.

In addition to academic challenges and struggles, interview participants also stated that relationship conflicts contributed to not-good days. Family members and friends played a large role in the students' lives, and they indicated it was a bad day when there were family arguments, friendship conflicts, or romantic struggles. Students talked about "personal conflicts" with sadness and emotion. A challenging day for Quinn included getting "in a fight with my parents." These arguments had their origins in their earlier years while living at home, and they continued when the student moved away to attend college. Other family conflicts did not just involve parents and children. For example, Robin may not be fighting with their parents, but a difficult day was when the parents fought with each other:

> In my first year [of] college, there was something that happened to my family. I came from Vietnam about 7 or 8 years ago, and there I was very much surrounded by my family. My mom and my dad didn't have any arguments very much, but when they came here, they [started] to have arguments almost every single day. That was when I was stressed, or things were stressful, and I was stressed at college. When I came home, and then I could hear them starting to make the argument, it started to affect me a lot.

Family relationships were not the only relationships that were important to college students. These students stated that friendships were also important in their lives. Cameron considered a challenging day when "something happened to a friend" or when "something terrible happened to a friend." Shannon was also vague about relationship issues:

> If any of the relationships in my life is having an issue, it can really make me feel down. I'm very connection-based, so if any of those connections feel bad, my whole day is off. Those are indicators of bad days.

Although interview participants did not go into specific details about relationship problems, they did highlight the importance of family and intimate relationships in their lives: "If I have an argument with my family or with my girlfriend, that also weighs on me. Even if I'm having a good day and then I have that one issue with my relationships can offset everything." The family was a source of conflict and pain for these college students. On a daily basis, it was a challenge to get along or coexist peacefully. Sometimes the conflicts go much deeper into the past. The accumulation of pain sometimes comes from the generations before and they get passed on to the current generation.

## Intergenerational Trauma

In the book *On Earth We're Briefly Gorgeous*, the author writes about the physical and sexual trauma his grandmother and mother went through and explains what it was like going through childhood in an abusive home. This epistolary novel describes his grandmother's life as a prostitute during the Vietnam War and giving birth to his mother, who also enters into abusive and violent relationships later in life. The author has noted that this novel was inspired by his own life experiences; he has stated in interviews that he sees himself as the protagonist in this novel. The novel chronicles the trauma that gets passed on from one generation to another as family members both rely on and fear each other.[3] The continuing intergenerational trauma is described by the college students I interviewed as they talked about their family background.

Participants referenced their family histories to explore and discuss their current psychological distress. These college students considered how trauma gets passed on from one generation to the next in "a vicious cycle." Trauma includes physical hardship and psychological pain, and Quinn stated that "a lot [of] mental health problems can also be genetics." In addition, participants suggested that if physical and psychological trauma were not addressed in one generation, they would get passed on to the next generation with devastating consequences. Evelyn stated that there were multiple suicide attempts on both sides of their family. They talked specifically about the destructive events from their mother's side of the family. For example, their maternal grandfather fought in the Korean War, and Evelyn speculated that he suffered from post-traumatic stress disorder due to his long-term exposure to brutality and violence. Furthermore, their maternal grandmother's younger brother died while she was carrying him on her back in cold and harsh conditions during the war. Evelyn believed that their mother's younger brother did not speak until he was much older because "there was definitely some trauma there." This collective family experience with violence and pain has a profoundly negative impact on three generations sharing the same household:

My grandparents, my mom's parents, don't speak to each other even though we live in the same house. They don't speak to each other because I'm assuming she's done with his abuse. And me realizing that he abused my mom and my grandma, it really messes with me because I love him. But I also know he's done terrible things, and his room is right across from mine. And I feel like everybody's waiting for him to die, but I've seen him as this grandfather figure, not the ugly side of him. So, that's just kind of hard to live with, I guess. And because of the things that both my parents went through, I feel like they want to be there for me emotionally. But it's not possible. It's just not possible for them because they haven't worked through their own trauma.

Whereas Evelyn elaborated on their parents' emotional unavailability, others speculated about lingering family trauma and its influence on parenting styles. Taylor reflected on living in a household with three generations and noticing their parents' style of raising children. They shared that intergenerational trauma impacted the way they were raised because "I do see, especially now that I'm living with my grandparents, how their perspectives have impacted the way my parents think and contribute to their parenting style."

Participants described the interactions between their grandparents and parents to better understand their own family upbringing and treatment. For example, grandparents did not communicate with parents in an emotionally supportive manner; in turn, parents did not communicate with their children in an emotionally supportive manner. In general, college students discussed how emotions were not part of the usual daily social interactions. Parents and children may talk about what they will be doing each day, but they did not share their emotions regarding these activities. In general, there were not conversations about personal feelings or emotions on either side. Children were not asked about their feelings or emotions by parents or grandparents. Jamie saw this in their own family. They discussed the parenting styles across two generations and growing up with limited emotional and mental health support:

> We have three generations in one household and, so, seeing the way that my grandparents interact with my parents, I could just tell that the dynamic of a mental health topic and conversation wasn't there because they don't really talk. It's more of this kind of dynamic where you know you're loved, so you don't need anything else. You know it, so you don't need to be treated too well. You don't need to be asked whether you're doing okay. You don't need to have that emotional support that a family usually is supposed to give when you're an adult because you can handle it on your own. That's kind of what I got from my grandparents talking to my parents, so my parents didn't treat me any differently from how they were treated.

The family structure reproduced limited emotional support in each generation. The participants were not encouraged to discuss their struggles with mental health challenges in the family environment. In addition to a lack of emotional support, some students also experienced physical violence in the home. For example, one form of physical violence was parents hitting their children. Cameron discussed the damaging impact of physical violence from past generations on the current and future generations. They explained that "parents unwillingly and unconsciously" pass on their parents' abusive behavior to their own children because they were abused as children. In other words, parents "don't know how to treat their kids properly because they've never been treated properly." Cameron further discussed the broader context of this behavior:

> In Asian American communities, violence is almost a social norm. You know, I'm laughing because, oh, I'm going to get hit by my parents, stuff like that. We Asian kids laugh about it. But if you look at it from a different cultural perspective, it's just like, "Whoa, your parents hit you. Is everything okay?" I feel like we're so desensitized to the point where it's become sort of like a stereotypical cultural norm. With Asian American parents, it's definitely a generational thing, for sure.

In some cases, participants emotionally talked about their parents' childhood struggles before they came to the United States. The physical and financial hardships were difficult for the students to imagine, and it left them with feelings of guilt and remorse for their parents' suffering. Although they are appreciative of their life in the United States, they are also burdened with the stories of their parents' difficult family life. Hayden explained these mixed feelings of sadness and gratitude:

> My dad grew up in the Philippines, and he didn't exactly have an easy life. He had a very hard life. I think he and his family were very poor. Whenever I go back to the Philippines, I can kind of see where he's coming from. So, I feel like, whenever he tells me about his life story, maybe in his mind I need to know where we came from to know that if I wasn't born or raised here in the U.S. and I ended up being born and raised in the Philippines, what my life could have been. But I feel like a lot of the time, that weighs on me because I know that I'll never be able to live the life that he went through. I have been told that I should be grateful for my life here.

The trauma that began in one generation and continued to the next negatively impacted the participants' developmental years. The students believed they received limited emotional support from their parents. They attributed this deficit to their parents' own family life experiences. However, Alex believed that there would be changes in their generation. They explained that their grandparents' and parents' generations were discouraged from showing emotional vulnerability, whereas their generation is learning to be comfortable with processing their emotions and expressing their feelings. Alex stated that intergenerational trauma may end in their generation: "I think my generation now is kind of like a turning point in a way. I mean, for me, I don't think I would be the same to my children." The trauma that connects multiple generations is related to the human need for spaces where they feel safe and protected. Feelings of security also come from feeling a sense of belonging in new and old surroundings.

## Thwarted Belongingness

A sense of belonging is vital to human survival. Individuals who lack a sense of belonging also lack a sense of place where they can achieve their life goals. Thwarted belongingness is the perception that one is isolated from others and does not form a vital part of a valued social group. An individual does not feel a sense of belonging because they lack positive interactions with a certain group of individuals in a caring environment.[4] Research in this area noted that one way to conceptualize the idea of belonging on campus is to examine an individual's view of whether they feel included in the campus community. This conceptualization of the sense of belonging is particularly useful when focusing on historically marginalized populations such as Asian American college students.[5] The current study found similarities from previous research which demonstrated that Asian American students perceive that they are not as fully integrated into the greater university community as European American students.[6]

Participants did not feel a sense a belonging on the college campus. Participants experienced thwarted belongingness through cultural adjustments and social expectations, academic challenges and imposter syndrome, and racial tensions and campus racism. The transition from high school to college was a period of cultural adjustment for participants. They were leaving the familiarity of high school to enter into an unfamiliar and uncertain community. They wondered if they would be able to make friends and adjust to their new surroundings. Many were leaving their high school friends behind because their friends did not choose college as a current pathway while others were heading to their own chosen college campuses. The anticipation and preparation for a college move were made more difficult for some college students because they were only children or the eldest children in their families. In these situations, the college student did not have a model to emulate or advice to follow. This made the college move more unpredictable and frightening. Robin stated that being the first child in their family to go to college was a confusing and solitary time:

> I didn't really know what to expect. I didn't have anyone to talk to me about what it would be like in college. When I first came to college, I didn't know what to do. I didn't know anyone here.

The university was a new place that was vastly different from what they were used to in their home communities. Students found that leaving home and going away to college was a lonely experience; at the same time, they found that coming back home also presented new cultural challenges. On the one hand, they were still trying to find their way in college. At the same time, they found that returning home was also difficult. They didn't fit in at college and they didn't fit in when they returned home. These movements involved adapting to cultural changes. Jamie found the need to constantly negotiate the new cultural spaces each time they came back home or went back to school:

> Some challenges that I faced as a college student was the pressure of assimilating in my community because I'm an Asian student who came from a very cultural background. It was quite difficult for me to not feel weird telling my friends at school about the habits I have that come from my family. Another challenge I faced was going back home. So, kind of having a culture shock coming here and then having a culture shock going home because, here, I'm a Chinese girl that knows a lot of Cantonese, and I'm very cultural in my ways. But then going back home, I'm very American, close to a White girl. I can't speak Cantonese to my grandparents in a very fluent way. I was trying to find the balance between my identity with my family as well as my identity with my college community.

The back and forth journey between home and school generated stress for students as they adjusted to two different homes during the college years. Some students found the campus space more challenging because they did not see themselves reflected in the university. Students talked about finding their cultural spaces over time as they acclimated to college life. Finding a place where they culturally belonged helped them feel more comfortable in college. Taylor stated, "I feel the most belonging when I'm with the Asian cultural organizations." Asian student organizations helped students feel a sense of belonging; it was a place where students could express their authentic multiple identities. Identifying with multiple identities meant that students did not find their full selves in any one particular social space. Rather, they had to look to multiple students organizations to find social connectedness. These student organizations were meaningful to students because they would identity with others who looked like them and shared common experiences. Kelly talked about the importance of advocating for the self by exploring the campus and finding an assortment of resources that were personally good fits. Although it was not always easy to find an organization or program that was a good fit for them, Kelly continued to research available resources and campus support. They finally found a program that focused on the mental health of Asian American college students which was sponsored by the university's psychological counseling services. Kelly talked about this protected and safe space:

> I think me being a marginalized student in multiple ways, identifying as a queer Asian American student. I didn't see myself reflected in the university a lot, and it's something that I had to continuously navigate. I did not see myself represented in all of my identities in any one place but finding spaces where I was at least represented in some way, shape, or form by faculty, peers, and through university programs. In those ways, I was able to navigate the university a little bit better. I was involved with a workshop program at school: the mental health and Asian-American–centered workshop program sponsored through counseling and psychological services. In that space, I was able to express my queer Asian identities as well as explore mental health in a constructive way.

Some students found a strong sense of belonging in more than one space. Students found places where they could grow and thrive in cultural groups and academic programs. For example, one student identified their Asian sorority as a comfortable cultural space as well as the nursing program, where there was a strong Asian student presence. Because the campus had a large student population, it was more meaningful to meet other college students in smaller communities. Being in smaller groups generated a greater sense of belonging for participants. The sense of belongingness was developed in these smaller groups through shared cultural experiences and academic goals. Therefore, the combination of small group interaction and shared identities and interests helped participants cultivate a sense of belonging. Dana discussed the spaces where they belonged on campus:

> I think that I actually have a pretty good sense of belonging. Being in the nursing program is a smaller community: about 140 people in my overall class. I do feel like I belong there. People want to be there, and they're my friends. I also think that after joining the sorority, I do have a support system of people who care about me. I think those instances of being in smaller groups helps me, like, feel like I belong. In the grand scheme of things, I did mention that there's a lot more White people versus Asian people on campus, so sometimes I just feel a little out of place, but it doesn't really contribute to my sense of belonging.

Although coming into a new cultural and social space as a college student presented challenges, over time, interviewees were able to find some places on campus where they could grow and thrive as students and as human beings. However, social expectations in college created a lot of physical and psychological stress for college students.

Most participants felt the pressures of social expectations at some point in their college years. For some, the pressures of social expectations were temporary and did not negatively impact their college studies. For others, these pressures were more prolonged and enduring as they tried to gain approval through peer interactions. Gaining approval was not easy and was often a competitive process because not every person who wanted a position in the membership was accepted. It was highly competitive to gain membership into student organizations and internships. The social expectations usually came from trying to participate in and gain acceptance into student organizations. Morgan felt this challenge when arriving in college:

> I think coming into college, there was always a pressure for me that I put on myself to kind of get involved. Whether that was when I joined a fraternity freshman year, it was something that was pressure I put on myself. To go meet these guys and make myself stand out in order for me to get noticed by these guys and end up joining the brotherhood. There was pressure to join other clubs. There's always pressure to do stuff. I also think that there's pressure to get internships.

The need to belong to student organizations and feel accepted by peers was a social challenge on campus. Finding a club or organization to join was one task; feeling accepted and appreciated in that student group was another challenge. In the same way that students were accepted into college and found the college experience challenging, students were accepted into student organizations and found the experience generally negative. There was a constant need to present and behave in socially expected ways. When students did not fulfill these social expectations from the student group, they did not enjoy belonging to that student organization. Shannon did not feel accepted by one student organization:

> I'm going to be really honest. There are some Filipino organizations on campus that I never felt connected with because the people who are in those organizations actually made me feel that I had to look a certain way in order to fit in. A huge thing was the way I dressed, the way I did my hair and my makeup. It really got down to that, so that was a big pressure. A big pressure was also being very much a people person. I don't know if I'm using the right term, but I honestly like to be social. That was a huge pressure. I felt like I always had to be on. I felt that way physically, and that was really a big pressure.

In addition to feeling the pressure to look a certain way in order to gain organizational approval, college students experienced other pressures and expectations. Some of these came from experiencing tremendous academic challenges. Participants felt academic pressures and challenges while in college. With regard to academics, participants communicated the importance of working hard and earning good grades as "non-negotiable." Earning good academic scores was a goal because they also had future plans for graduate school or professional school. Taylor explained their long-term professional goals and the need to focus on their undergraduate studies: "I do plan to go to med school, so there is a lot of pressure of doing well in academics." Several expressed the competitive atmosphere of reaching academic excellence and found they needed to perform to the best of their ability. Evelyn stated their motivation to do well in school: "I'm very competitive." Students expressed the importance of their academic journey. Table 1.1 shows the participants' majors, minors, and emphases.

Table 1.1 Participants and Their Majors, Minors, and Emphases

| Participant | Major, Minor, and Emphasis |
| --- | --- |
| Alex | Nursing |
| Cameron | International business with an emphasis on Japanese |
| Dana | Nursing |
| Evelyn | Kinesiology |
| Hayden | Moving in the direction of occupational therapy |
| Jamie | Criminal justice, psychology, and social work |
| Kelly | Journalism and psychology |
| Morgan | Communications major and Spanish minor |
| Quinn | Kinesiology |
| Robin | Art, sociology, and women's studies |
| Shannon | Sociology major and leadership minor |
| Taylor | Biology |

Although the scholastic pressures were evident throughout their years in college, some students discussed the specific challenges in the earlier years of college life. They highlighted the first year of college as particularly difficult and challenging. There were adjustments and adaptations in their lives. In particular, they discussed the academic challenges in that first year. Hayden highlighted the continuing academic challenges that started in the first year of college:

> I feel like throughout my college career, I've played the catch-up game. The first time I played it was my first year, and it was really terrible because I didn't do well my first semester in college, and then I tried re-taking classes that I had previously failed into that spring semester, and it turned out to be so overwhelming that it made my situation even worse.

Whereas Hayden expressed the ongoing frustration with this never-ending cycle of academic stress, some pointed to not understanding how the college system operated as they tried to work on their educational goals. The students discussed their educational ambitions and aspirations; however, they did not always receive the assistance they needed to reach their educational objectives. Kelly discussed how their perfectionist tendencies to aim for academic excellence led to choosing two majors of study. However, they explained the challenges of moving around the different academic departments within this bureaucratic maze:

> Early on, I knew that I wanted to pursue a double major, which immediately meant more classes and navigating the university differently because, academically, I didn't have the same tools to navigate the differences in curriculum requirements. And then also adding a minor on top of that. It was a lot of pressure, and I admit I put myself in that situation. I found it difficult to navigate how to choose classes in an order that made sense to remain on track to graduate. Within the institution, I didn't find a centralized place, so I had to go to different departments, clarifying and asking questions and really putting in the effort to ensure that I was on track to do what I wanted to do, but the university didn't always provide the tools to make that easier.

The aim for academic excellence was a demanding and stressful process for participants. There was added pressure when they saw other students do well in classes while they were struggling. One student articulated this sense of academic competition: "I'm seeing all these accomplishments of everyone else. We're all trying to do the same thing, but you're already doing this. What was I doing? Why didn't I do that?" These feelings of doubt impacted the students' sense of belonging in the academic world. They felt like an imposter in this new academic setting. Research has shown that many intelligent and capable individuals, particularly college students, believe that their current success is due to luck, and they fear that they will be exposed as imposters or frauds.[7] Two college students discussed their feelings with imposter syndrome to explain their lack of belonging in college. They questioned their academic abilities and wondered if they truly belonged at the university or college. Dana talked about the culture of academic competition among students in the nursing program:

> In group chats, sometimes, they stress me out a lot because they're talking about an exam that's 2 weeks out, and I can't think about this right now. There is that kind of academic pressure because I'm hard on myself. I want to do the best that I can. I want to do well on tests and everything, but that doesn't always happen, so that makes me nervous and puts pressure on me. Another source of pressure is just keeping up with everybody. Just having imposter syndrome as a college student or a nursing student. I definitely feel that they're studying so much more than me. I need to be doing this and that because they're doing it. I try to tell myself that I have my own way of doing things.

The feeling of not belonging on the college campus also came from not living in the campus residential spaces. Students living off-campus did not believe they were receiving the ideal college experience because they felt left out of the on-campus social activities. This separated them from other students who were engaged in residential activities. Off-campus students did not feel like they were getting the full college experience. In turn, they did not feel connected to the campus as a whole. This lack of connection to the campus made them not feel a sense of belonging to the college culture. They felt like impostors or frauds. The feelings of being a fraud were overwhelming for Shannon because they did not feel a sense of academic or social belonging:

The first year was so tough because I didn't live on campus, and everyone's posting on their social media how much fun they're having or the connections they're making. It didn't help that during rush week all the fraternities and sororities are out and seeing how selective they were in who they wanted to talk to. It definitely felt like I had this imposter syndrome. I was like, "Why am I even in college?" Obviously, I'm not succeeding. I was not a 4.0 student. What am I doing here? Why am I wasting someone's spot? I was questioning my own abilities, which unfortunately deteriorated and affected my GPA. I think it was my lowest GPA ever. It was really sad because it was my first year, and I was really trying to find my way. I don't even know how I got from there to here. It was definitely hard.

In addition to academic challenges, college students also experienced social challenges. They discussed their social interactions with the overall college population and described their negative experiences interacting with people who did not belong to their race. In this study, all participants had a story to share about race. Several students stated that they experienced personal racism in college; four indicated they did not experience personal racism but that the perceived racism was more indirect. One student was not sure if they experienced personal racism or indirect racism. Students saw indirect racism as a campus problem. Hayden and Shannon spoke specifically about the racist statements that came out at a Zoom meeting at the beginning of the global pandemic. Hayden was a member of this cultural student group, whereas Shannon was not; however, they stated, "Although I am not a part of this student organization, that doesn't mean I don't support the group." The Zoom meeting was interrupted by a non-member who made hurtful racist statements to the members of this student group. Although Hayden and Shannon were not in attendance during this racist disruption, they were deeply saddened and upset that this happened in a protected space. Hayden expressed their feelings about this particular event:

> My student organization was having their elections for the board. I was planning on attending, but I actually didn't go, but I think a lot of us within the college community saw the result of how one or two people—I think just one—Zoom bombed our meeting, and they said something along the lines of "Do you all have coronavirus?" Since we're all Asian, we took that to heart, and we were very upset as a community, not just for Filipinos but for Asians in general. We were really upset over that.

Research has shown that since the coronavirus was first reported in China, people of Asian descent have been treated as scapegoats based solely on their race.[8] For example, Stop AAPI Hate, a national coalition that became the authority on gathering data on racially motivated attacks related to the pandemic, received 4,548 incident reports in 2020 and 4,533 incident reports in 2021.[9] College students discussed some of these experiences while they were still on campus before moving to remote learning. One student also talked about a particular racist incident at the beginning of the global pandemic and the lingering effects of this experience:

> There was actually a time when the COVID cases started coming up, and someone asked me if I eat bat. I think that was the most directly disrespectful comment I ever got being a Chinese woman. I had never previously experienced that because the high school I went to was always populated with Chinese Americans. So, having that asked to me just put a bad taste in my mouth. I knew that type of racism was out there, but it's just really infuriating when it happens to you, personally, because you can only understand it to a certain extent when you see it happening [to] other people, and you can

be empathetic. You can try your best to understand, but you don't really understand the anger that comes with it until you experience it yourself.

Students experienced perceived racism even before the start of the global pandemic. Participants also shared their feelings about perceived racism in the physical classroom spaces. They articulated that these experiences were particularly disturbing because they were in college to learn and to earn their degrees. Most of the waking hours were spent in the classroom. Although this was not Taylor's personal experience, they discussed how their friends were made to feel uncomfortable with the racial language that professors and students used in the classroom:

> I would say a lot of the times it happens in the classroom. It would be like something that another student said during a discussion or something, and it's blatantly racist. My friend would be speaking up about it, but then it would just come back with more aggressive— what is it, I guess—backlash standing up to it. I know professors have said a couple comments that made them uncomfortable. But then, in that situation, my friend didn't feel they were able to do anything because it wasn't really relevant to the discussion, but it was still blatantly racism.

Taylor specifically stated that they did not want to go into further details. On the other hand, another student stated that they have never experienced racism in college. Rather, Morgan contrasted Taylor's explanation of blatant racism in the classroom with what they called "friendly banter between people" outside of the classroom. Whereas Taylor focused on the classroom experience, Morgan focused on a non-classroom experience to discuss race.

Morgan explained the context of this experience as interaction with their friends:

> I wouldn't consider it as blatant racism. Everybody experiences the racist jokes. I would say pretty much my entire college experience, there have been a few amount of Asians compared to White people, so I get the small eyes joke or the Asian joke, but I don't consider that as racism. Everyone has their own set of humor when it comes to their friend groups. They might poke fun at Asians, and I'll say a White joke, and we'll laugh. I mean, I'm half White and half Asian. I look more Asian, but I wouldn't consider anything as racism. Obviously, there's a line to be drawn. I haven't hit that line. None of my friends have ever hit that line, and none of my friends would ever stand for anything that crosses that line.

In addition to the classroom spaces, participants did not experience a welcoming environment around the open campus spaces. Robin did not feel a sense of belonging inside and outside of the classroom. Although words were not directed at them, they felt isolated and ignored by classmates and other college students:

> I feel the most bad when I'm taking the class, and there are no Asian people in there. I feel that the person who is different from me would pick a person who is similar to them to talk to because they have good English skills while they ignore me, a person who is different than them who has dark hair and who doesn't speak a lot. When I walk around on campus, and the person is in an organization, they will pick the person who has blond hair or blue eyes to talk to them about the organization: Do you want to join? Do you have any concerns about this? They will not pick a person like me who is standing next to them, so that's when I feel I experienced racism: when I am overlooked.

The Asian American students found that they made up a small percentage of the college population. These small numbers are noticeable to college students and they are not sure what these numbers mean in the larger scheme of things. Although these small numbers do not indicate that there is racism in the Greek system, it is a contributing question to wonder if racism has something to do with the lower numbers. For example, Alex discussed their experiences in the Greek system in which there were few Asian student members in a predominantly White sorority:

> I don't know if this is like a racist thing, but I'm in a sorority, and I think out of like a hundred people in my class that joined, there's probably like three or four Asian girls. So, that was kind of something else.

By contrast, Dana talked about their experiences in a predominantly Asian sorority by describing how the members are stereotyped as "really pretty" because they have "dyed hair, painted nails, tattoos, wear a lot makeup, and drink heavily." Dana further explained that people who are not Asian are attracted to this type of person:

> In general, since there's not a big Asian population at this school, when I walk around campus, it felt like there weren't that many people who looked like me, which is definitely a shock from high school because there's a lot of Asian people there. I've never been super worried about fitting in, but it was just a switch. There have been comments, just smaller comments about yellow fever, that kind of thing. A lot of generalizations about me being in an Asian sorority and just a big stereotype. But to my knowledge, I haven't really experienced really bad behaviors and stuff.

A lack of Asian student presence was also evident in other social organizations, including membership on the cheerleading team. Evelyn elaborated on their interaction with the other team members by focusing on their conversations about academic achievement. The team members believed Evelyn had excellent grades, even though that was not necessarily the case. Quinn shared similar experiences with the false assumption of high-achieving Asians:

> I feel like there's a stereotype with Asians that we're overachieving and are just generally smarter, which I don't find true all the time. I feel like sometimes my teachers have expected more out of me just because I'm Korean.

In Evelyn's case, there was the perception that Evelyn was very smart because they were Asian and, therefore, would be available for tutoring services. According to Evelyn, these academic assumptions and expectations were examples of racial microaggressions:

> If you look at the cheerleading team, it's dominantly White. I may be getting an A in a class, and that's the expectation. I get that a lot from my teammates. Just assumptions that I'm smarter than them, which may be true, but it was just off-putting. And just not being able to relate to a lot of them because I came from a more culturally diverse area back home. It was just these small microaggressions. I've had a lot of friends coming at me for tutoring, and oftentimes, I would be able to help them. But people would just assume that I would be good in every subject. English is not a strong suit for me at all, and friends would come to me: "Can you proofread this?" I'm struggling to maintain a B plus in my comp and writing class. I don't know if you want my advice.

Hayden also shared their experiences with racial microaggressions at a student organization function dedicated to collecting donations and supplies for those experiencing food insecurity:

> There was one moment, [and] this might be just a microaggression. I was volunteering to collect food supplies. I was having a conversation with this person who was White, and his friend who was also White came up to us and started talking with his friend. This person who just came didn't even look at me. He was not making any eye contact with me, just trying to filter me out of the conversation not rudely but with his body language. I think that's the extent of what I've experienced with racism.

Although words were not directed at Hayden, there was still the sense that he was rendered invisible during this short social interaction. Racial microaggressions refer to "brief and commonplace daily verbal, behavioral, and environmental indignities, whether intentional or unintentional, that communicate hostile, derogatory, or negative racial slights and insults to the target person or group."[10] Racial microaggressions occur on an interpersonal level, including among one's peers.[11] Race scholars have challenged the term "racial microaggression" because it minimizes the psychological harm that comes from daily and persistent mistreatment; they prefer the term "racist abuse" because it highlights the profound negative effects on the targeted individual, including distress, anger, worry, depression, anxiety, pain, fatigue, and suicide.[12] These are all examples of trauma, which generates prolonged hopelessness and pain.[13]

In other campus spaces, the social interaction was prolonged and extended. For example, participants discussed their experiences living with roommates. Students described how they did not feel comfortable around their roommates due to differences in music preferences or food choices. Jamie explained that their roommates told them to turn off the music when they played Chinese music because it sounded foreign to them, and the roommates also made negative comments about their food choices. These negative social interactions made Jamie feel protective of and defensive about their cultural background:

> I had a few encounters where simple things that are very popular like house slippers or eating certain foods weirded out the people that I met in college. For example, I tell them about dim sum, which is very different from what people eat if they're not Asian. I've had some small conversations that I noticed were kind of like backhanded compliments: "I'll eat your food, but don't tell me what's in it. Don't tell me what it is." And I'm like, okay. I felt like that was a very stereotypical answer. Just because we have a different type of meal doesn't mean I'm going to feed you something that's not safe for you to eat. It kind of made me feel a little bit more reserved about my culture, like I kind of wanted to defend it.

This example highlights how Asian American college students are made to feel different from their peers; it is a reminder that these cultural differences are not accepted in mainstream society. Asian Americans experience prejudice and discrimination in a unique way compared to other racial and ethnic groups in the United States, as they are often perceived as perpetual foreigners or aliens.[14] Research has shown that this form of racial prejudice and discrimination is associated with negative mental outcomes, including depression, anxiety, substance abuse, and suicide ideation. One study demonstrated that the perpetual foreigner label placed an individual from the farthest point of being an insider. Thus, labeled individuals experienced feelings of inferiority as outsiders.[15] Furthermore, thwarted belongingness, in the form of the perpetual foreigner myth, was a significant risk factor for suicide ideation among Asian American and Asian international college students.[16]

On a different scale, students discussed the broader context of racism, including the model minority myth. The term "model minority" has been used to describe how some educators explained the rising academic, professional, and financial success of Asian Americans in the United States. Asian Americans' overall success indicated that they had fulfilled the American Dream of fitting into American society and achieving material success despite their perceived differences from the dominant culture.[17] Furthermore, the model minority stereotype reflects the view that Asian Americans are more successful academically, economically, and socially compared with other racial minority groups in the United States due to the emphasis on hard work and a belief in meritocracy. Asian Americans who do not live up to the model minority standard experience negative mental health outcomes.[18]

Kelly articulated that although they did not experience racism in a personal way, they have come to understand that the model minority myth is a contributing factor in institutional racism, which played a part in the lack of an Asian American Studies major at this particular college:

> Nothing sticks out in my mind about experiencing a racist moment, but from an institutional standpoint, I will say I felt it a lot. As I grew in my college studies, I learned a lot about institutional racism and

the way that affects students without us realizing it or knowing it. Asian Americans are seen as the model minority and are not served as much as other ethnic minorities. This has been a disservice to me and my peers as Asian American Pacific Islander students. We don't have an Asian American Studies program, whereas we do have a Chicano Studies program. We have an Africana Studies program and other ethnic minority studies, but we don't have one currently for Asian Americans. As a result, I haven't been able to feel as connected to my heritage through the university and through academics as much as other people might.

Throughout the years, the model minority myth meaning has transformed, and it has highlighted how Asian Americans do not belong in the United States. For example, Asian American college students struggle with feelings of isolation on campus because there is a perceived separation between racial groups; these feelings of isolation contribute to feelings of embarrassment, shame, and depression. In addition, researchers have identified feelings of embarrassment and shame as major stressors for Asian American college students.[19]

One student discussed the culture of races and spaces on the college campus. There was the broader context of racism in the United States that was perpetuated on campus. Cameron and a friend noticed that White students did not share the campus space with non-White students. For example, Cameron's Asian friend would walk around campus and found that White students would not move out of their way and the groups would end up running into each other; however, when they walked in the path of non-White students, the students of color would move away, allowing Cameron's friend to safely pass. Cameron focused on one's family upbringing to explain why some students did not yield campus spaces while others did:

> I believe it's the way White people are brought up, not to say that it's a bad thing. We concluded that upbringing, in general, is very different. I feel like a lot of Asian American people are taught to always respect other people, to look out for other people, to be attentive to other people that they kind of lose themselves because they're so into the idea of appeasing other people. But at the end of the day, you have to care for yourself, as well.

## Perceived Burdensomeness

The path to adult independence often begins in the college years. Individuals thrive when they are able to use their abilities and skills to solve problems. There is a general sense that college students do not want to be troublesome or an inconvenience to other people. For example, Shannon did not want to be a disappointment to others by asking for help: "I feel like a burden having to ask for help." Perceived burdensomeness refers to the perception that one is a burden to family members, friends, and/or society; the individual believes that personal flaws become a social liability.[20] In our interviews, participants stated they had been a burden to someone at some point in their lives. They felt that they were now in college and should be able to manage their own lives and solve their own problems. Jamie expressed the feelings of learning to gain more independence and relying on their own resources:

> I do feel as though I am a burden when I talk to people about my problems or if I can't do something on my own and I have to ask for help. That's usually when I feel like a burden because I have a

predisposed notion that I have to figure things out on my own 100% of the time.

The main people they are a burden to are family members and close friends. There was the perception that they were a financial burden to their parents as they pursued their college education. Students also talked about feeling a burden to their friends when they overshared information or relied on them too much for mental support.

Participants discussed family concerns and responsibilities as added college pressures. One source of family tension was attending college far away from home. Several participants lived in other states from their home families, and others were several hours' drive away from home. While college students were adjusting to the new norms of being a college student far away from home, they also embraced their identities as someone's child far from home. This meant that while they were trying to excel in their studies, they also often thought about their family members. Being far away from their families meant that sometimes the college students worried about their parents and younger siblings back home. These thoughts required time and energy in an already busy academic life. Evelyn lived a distance from their family and frequently worried about their mother's physical health:

> My mom is chronically ill. I was living in one city, and I'd be worried because she's all the way in another city. I could drive there, but she's still far away. I'd be worried about her health. She's had strokes and all these other health issues. So, it was something sitting in the back of my head: Is my mom doing okay? Is my sister doing okay? How's my family doing? So just thinking about my family a lot.

At the same time, college students were also aware that their family thought about them, too. This in turn generated some feelings of guilt. They were not comfortable with the thought that their parents were worrying about them. The geographical distance was hard on the college student, and knowing that it was also hard on the family members back home made it an overwhelming thought process for the college student each day. Evelyn also discussed feeling like a burden to their parents: "I just feel like a burden to my family, mostly. I feel like I'm wasting their time. I feel like they worry a lot about me. Emotionally, I am a burden to them."

Some college students lived closer to their family home, and some lived in the family home while attending college. Family responsibilities were more active for these students compared to those living far away from home, and they sometimes found the need to balance academic work and family obligations. Some of these family responsibilities included taking care of younger siblings in the home while also learning how to develop their own independence as college students. However, learning to become more independent was a lonesome experience for the college students because they could not talk to their parents or their younger siblings about their own college struggles. Robin explained the stress of living at home while focusing on the demands of their college courses and taking care of their younger siblings. In addition, there were daily tensions between their father and mother:

> My parents were making an argument every day in college, and I cannot talk to anyone because my parents expect me to be independent. Even though if I try to talk to them, they maybe will not

understand me because they were inside themselves, and they expect me to grow up and be independent. I have to look after my little sister and my little brother, and they very much depend on me, so I can't talk to them about college stress. I worry if I talk to them like this that they will stay away from college because of my college experience. It's very stressful for me to be a college student, especially as the first person to go to college. I get stress from the family. I get pressure from the family.

Furthermore, while the participants were not able to share their academic challenges with their family members, they also did not want to disappoint their parents. There was an added weight when the students compared themselves to other high academic achieving family members and did not want to fail in their studies. Shannon wanted to succeed academically like their father and sister:

My family values education a lot. Education is very huge in my family. My dad has his master's degree and a bachelor's degree. My sister is getting her master's degree. There is a lot of familial pressure, which I internalized during freshman year of college. I have a lot of big shoes to fill from people who came before me.

Similarly, participants looked up to their older siblings and did not want to disappoint their family. They felt the need to aspire to the same level of accomplishment set by family members. Alex found that there were high expectations in her family to achieve in the field of medicine:

My parents have really high expectations, and my older brother has been so successful. I feel like going into college, I have a lot of goals, and I feel like I have some big shoes to fill. I feel like I have to perform well to make my parents proud. I mean, no matter what, I just want my parents to be happy for me or be proud of me. And I don't want to let anyone down. Obviously, I want to set a good example for my little brother, who's only a year younger, but I feel he looks up to me and how I do things. Also, just being in nursing, it's already like there's a lot of comparison. I just want to do the best I can.

College students talked about doing the best they could in their studies but it just did not feel like enough, especially when they felt that their parents were comparing them to the more successful child in the family. Some participants felt that they were not as perfect as their siblings. Quinn talked about how they are different from their older sister who spent most of her time not socializing with friends:

> My sister and I are not close. I guess you could say that my sister was the favorite between the two of us. She didn't really spend a lot of time with her friends. I think honestly that she didn't have that many friends throughout high school and so she didn't go out that much which was something that my mom liked about her. This was confusing to me because I can't imagine a situation when you would want to see your child antisocial and depressed. My mom liked that about my sister so there's always been this underlying competition between the two of us.

To further understand this preferred child status, Quinn earlier discussed a bit about her mother's earlier life:

> My mom—I don't really hear a lot about the way she was raised. It seemed like she had a pretty good relationship with her parents. She always talks about how she spent all her time around my age just studying and never enjoying anything. She said that she started enjoying life in her late 40s. She never spent time with her friends

because her life was so based on being a complete workaholic. She always says "Oh, I didn't get to enjoy my life until later" which I feel is ridiculous. I feel like that's not something she should be proud of. I feel like my mom sees life as just working hard. I guess that's a generational thing.

In this situation, the perfect—and preferred—child was the one more like the mother.

In other words, working hard was the ideal characteristic in a child. Working hard was one way to please parents as students aimed to be perfect in their parents' eyes. Perfectionism was an emerging factor for suicide ideation among Asian American college students. The research found that the aim for perfectionism was a strong predictor for suicide ideation above and beyond feelings of hopelessness and depression.[21]

On the other hand, college students found that examining their parents' or siblings' academic history was useful when considering their own life goals. Participants found that looking to family members provided a frame of reference for them to think about their own professional goals. However, the conflicts emerged when parents and children did not see the value of particular majors or career paths in the same way. Some college students believed that their parents wanted them to excel in particular areas and did not see the merit in other majors or disciplines. In this way, the college students felt that they had limited choices by which to please their parents. Sometimes, these limited choices were not embraced by the college student, and problems arose when the student could not convey the value of their chosen major. The college student felt that the parents did not understand them or appreciate their own academic viewpoints. Jamie discussed how their mother did not understand their academic direction:

I have told my mom that I wanted to go into psychology or social work, any realm of helping people who don't have the resources that they need. And in my mom's eyes, mental health isn't really a problem. She kind of brushes it off like everyone should be fine. But if you do have mental problems, then you're weird. And you need to go to a hospital, something's wrong with you, and this isn't how it's supposed to be. So, in regards to my major, that's the push and pull between what I wanted to do, to help people who have mental health issues. And my mom's is kind of totally ignoring that mental health is part of my ambition.

Asian American college students negotiate personal, parental, and societal expectations. For example, students experience tremendous parental pressure to study diligently and to receive excellent grades. The participants in one study indicated that they were pressured to live by family values, including choosing certain majors and finding highly lucrative jobs.[22]

One participant talked about their siblings in another capacity. Sometimes, college students found that they could talk with their siblings in ways that they could not talk with their parents. In some of these conversations, college students conveyed their personal and academic problems in college. Thus, participants saw their siblings as allies and confidants. However, this type of relationship also produced feelings of guilt for the college students, particularly when they felt that they were oversharing their problems with their siblings. Taylor did not feel competition with their siblings, but they were concerned about overburdening their siblings with their personal and academic problems. They were also concerned about undue pressures on their siblings due to sibling comparison and evaluation:

I would say I probably feel the most burdensome to my siblings. I have learned not to rely or depend on too many friends because

I feel that since we are all stressed out, I shouldn't stress them out more when I talk to them. So, I kind of delegated all of my venting sessions and all of my emotions to my siblings. Of course, it's reciprocal. I listened to literally everything they share, but I do feel that I am the only one who is interested in medicine, and that is something that my family really appreciates. I don't want them to be compared to me, but it happens anyways.

College students understood the costly expenses that come with earning a 4-year degree. Financial concerns added to family tensions. Money issues created stress because interviewees relied on their parents' financial support to accomplish their academic goals. Alex stated it in this way: "In college, I feel like I'm a financial burden on my parents." One student felt like a financial burden when "my mom started holding my tuition over my head a lot. That was a big point of stress for me." Students expressed feelings of being a financial burden to their parents because they were taking too long to graduate. Although they understood that earning a college degree would take several years, they also felt that they were a financial drain on their family's resources: "I am definitely a financial burden to my parents." Evelyn is working on finding the balance between accepting their parents' financial support and understanding that academic work takes time:

> I've always felt like a burden, especially leading up to my attempt. I just felt like I was sucking all my parents' savings, wasting my time in school because I was not going fast enough. I felt like I was wasting my time, wasting everybody's time. I just felt like the biggest burden. I still do, to some degree, but I'm trying to work through that.

Financial considerations were also a concern for students who came to this college campus from another state. In addition to paying out-of-state tuition, the family also needed to consider traveling expenses to and from the college. There were also the usual financial costs associated with housing, books, and other campus fees. Alex explained the academic pressures they faced because their parents were paying out-of-state tuition for a public university:

> My parents are always on me about grades, and that's the main point because financially, I'm paying out-of-state tuition. I feel like I cannot take for granted that they can afford to send me here to do a nursing program. I don't want to put that money to waste. So, I want to make sure they get their money's worth.

Thus, college students felt the pressures to succeed and not fail in their classes because their parents were spending a lot of money for their college education. The research on perceived burdensomeness demonstrated that Asian American students experience great parental expectations for high academic achievement; consequently, these students may experience parental criticism, guilt, or shame when they underperform academically.[23] Participants considered the weight of their college education costs in other family situations. They discussed the need to be particularly diligent with their academic work; however, they also explained that the hard work they put into each day was generally not enough to their parents' satisfaction. College students felt the weight of their parents' negative evaluation of their academic efforts, often feeling that they needed to continuously study each day. They felt that their parents did not understand the necessity of free time to give the brain a rest. Quinn, another out-of-state student, explained that their mother's work ethic scrutiny made them feel less deserving of the family's financial support:

Let's say my mom doesn't see me studying one day or she catches me in my room watching TV. She'll be super upset with me because even if it's just me time and I did do work that day, she'll think that I'm just being lazy. She'll say, "Then what am I paying your tuition for?" And that makes me feel like I'm not doing enough.

Asian American college students who experienced high expectations for academic excellence also suffered mental health concerns, including depression and alienation. Researchers studied 292 Asian American undergraduate and graduate students at a medium-sized university in California and found that many Asian cultures have collectivist values that include unrealistic and perfectionist demands regarding academic achievement. These stresses and pressures place these students at risk for academic burnout as they aim for perfectionism.[24]

Some students were receiving financial aid. However, even with financial assistance, there was still the pressure to excel academically because the financial aid was made possible due to the parents' employment. In addition, receiving financial aid that was awarded due to their parents' history of work further added to students' guilt and growing sense of being a burden. For example, Hayden explained that even though they are receiving a tuition fee waiver due to their parent's employment, there was still the obligation to show appreciation to their father by proving that they are academically worthy of being a college student:

My dad is a veteran in the U.S. Navy. He served for 20 years and, due to his service, he was able to get this fee waiver benefit where all my tuition is paid off except for books or housing if I were to live on campus. It helps the family a lot, and it's a big load off my shoulders and my family's shoulders, but I feel like there's extra pressure to really excel and complete my college education because I have this big help. I'm going to grad school with those same benefits, and that's just extra pressure to continue excelling after I'm done with my bachelor's education. I'm going to be using my dad's benefits for my advantage, and I have to honor that with what I do.

Shannon received a similar tuition fee waiver but still felt like "a financial burden to have to ask my parents to help me pay for other fees because I also had a job at that time." Students expressed the financial cost of college and that even with a job they still sometimes needed their parents' financial support. Financial independence was also a challenge for college students.

In addition to considering the financial costs of education, there were also the daily costs of paying for food and housing. A few college students were not living with their parents and lived a more financially independent life from their families. Cameron talked about feeling financially insecure after experiencing almost homelessness:

> I'm not exactly the worst off, financially speaking, as evidenced by this roof over my head. I think that's a very narrow bridge to cross, though, because there were times where, truth be told, I almost experienced homelessness. Back in my freshman year of college, being financially stable as your center point could be very fragile. When that's gone, you don't really have anything to stand on.

Perceived burdensomeness might be a significant suicidal risk factor for some Asian American college students. Many Asian American communities share cultural norms that value maintaining family relationships and group cohesion. Therefore, the perception that one is a burden to one's family unit might be particularly devastating for Asian Americans.[25]

College students explained that they sometimes felt like a burden to their friends. Participants discussed the importance of being available to their friends in their time of need; however, there was also the concern that sometimes they were putting too much pressure on their friends to be available to them. They expressed a willingness to listen to their friends' problems but experienced feelings of guilt when they believed they were burdening their friends with their own problems. Therefore, the grace and patience they allowed for their friends were not perceived to apply to them. For example, Quinn understood that their friends might be emotionally exhausted from listening to their problems: "Sometimes, if I've been radiating negative energy for too long like from school stress or personal stress, I feel like it might be too much for my friends." In turn, this led to participants feeling guilty about sharing too much information about their personal challenges, including mental health struggles. College students felt that they were overburdening and overwhelming their friends with information that was too depressing. They believed that they were not being considerate of their friends' energy and time. Kelly expressed feelings of wasting their close friends' energy and time:

> I talk about it a lot with friends when I talk about my mental health struggles. It's something that I've been trying to learn not to feel. Throughout the years that I have shared with my close friends, there's always that sense of feeling like I'm a burden or feel guilt after the fact. I understand that they're coming from a place of concern and empathy, but I still sometimes can't help but feel like I'm sorry that I'm bothering them or that I'm wasting their time, or that I'm adding more negative energy into our friendship when that's not all our friendship is about.

College students also felt that their friendships were compromised when they asked too much of their friends. They believed that friendships were fragile and that they needed constant nurturing.

Asking friends for "comfort, advice, food, or money" did not make participants feel comfortable. Although they needed physical and emotional support, they also found that they did not want to burden their friends. Cameron explained that the most difficult human need to ask for was comfort:

> When I have to ask for something, whether it be a favor or anything for that matter, I guess. But I feel like a commonality for people who face, you know, mental illness is the idea that they don't want to be a burden. And that might amplify the emotion further, and I think that also speaks for myself as well when there are certain situations where I could have asked for help. And, quite frankly, I should have asked for help, but I didn't because of this fear of being a burden to someone else.

Sometimes when the participants felt that they overburdened their friends with information, they found that friends will tune them out. When the college students tried to share stories of their hardship and pain, they hoped that their friends would listen and provide emotional support; however, they sometimes felt that their friends were no longer paying attention. This made them feel as if they were talking to themselves or to a wall. Here is Jamie's story:

> I have a friend who I went to work some of my problems in my relationships. I felt like a burden when I was being brushed off because I know that some people just don't want to be like a bad person, and they know that when someone's opening up to them. It's kind of hard to just be like, "No, I don't want to do that." So,

I felt kind of like a burden that I wasn't exactly being listened to anymore. It was just more like me venting to a wall.

Suicidal thoughts and behaviors persisted throughout the college years. The accumulated pressures with cultural adjustments, social expectations, and academic pressures generated ongoing feelings of perceived burdensomeness, hopelessness, and depression. In addition, experiences with racial tensions and campus racism enhanced feelings of thwarted belongingness. Although the early college years were an exciting time to explore academic and social opportunities, they were also a period of feeling exhausted with continuing assignments, projects, and meetings. College students expressed the academic difficulties of having a heavy course load, looming deadlines, and not enough sleep. They believed that they were constantly working without a lot of leisure and recreation time. Many expressed that this constant treadmill of all work and no play was not sustainable. Taylor discussed experiencing burnout in the early college years:

> I never really understood what burnout meant until the second year. I think it was an accumulation of the very conflicting events such as dropping grades and additional opportunities that I didn't want to let go of, so I said yes. With a new position comes great expectations that need to be met, so that was also quite a burden.

Even when students worked hard, they did not always see the fruits of their labor. Although many worked very hard and remained dedicated to their studies, their grades did not always represent their diligent hard work. Students expressed a sense of powerlessness with not being able to better their academic record. Over time, they learned that some of their friends were not doing well in school either. This information produced a strong sense of discouragement because it seemed impossible to be a scholar in good standing. They also saw that others around them were going through similar experiences with declining grades. This collective sharing about failing grades among friends was significant because these students believed that being removed from the university was inevitable.

In addition to academic pressures in college, there were also financial problems at home. College students understood that a college education was costly and that their parents were making tremendous sacrifices for them to go to college; thus, when they were not earning good grades, they felt guilty for wasting their parents' money. Sometimes, college students relied on other extended family members for financial support, and this furthered the guilt they experienced. These multiple academic and financial challenges generated feelings of hopelessness. Robin attributed their breaking point to the heavy burden of academic failures and financial hardships:

> I cannot fix my GPA. I was getting very bad grades. I was experiencing stress with my grades and my family, so I felt at that time I cannot live this life anymore. There was too much stress at the time. At the end of the day, I can't change my GPA, and that's when I feel like I don't belong in college. Everyone in college is getting a high GPA, and they are successful. I cannot talk to anyone, and I keep to myself. It is this time that I feel I have to end my life. I wanted to end this situation. During this time, my family was in financial need very much. My aunt and uncle help out my family a lot. Every year, we have to pay the money back to them because they let us borrow the money. At this time, I feel very stressful because after we didn't have money in the accounts. That was very stressful for my family and myself, so I had the idea of suicide at that time.

Occurrences with psychological vulnerability left a lasting negative impact on college students. Recalling a specific painful episode was difficult and disturbing for the participants. In the process of sharing their stories, college students spoke slowly as they tried to recollect the exact details of their emotional state that led to suicide ideation. Dana expressed their suicidal tendencies as thoughts without action:

> I've never gotten to the point where I like felt like I'm going to take action, like suicidal stuff. But there have been times. I don't really remember these that well because I kind of don't want to remember them. Sometimes, at home, I go to the pill cabinet, and I just look at the pills. I wouldn't touch anything. I wouldn't attempt to do anything, but I just think about it and know that the options are there.

Shannon described a particular moment of not being able to register for fall classes as a trigger that flashed back to earlier academic failures. They described their suicidal thoughts as falling into a hole; these feelings were so devastatingly powerful that they did not think they would live through another season:

> I vividly remember I was freaking out in my head, but physically you couldn't even tell that I was freaking out. I'm in a hole, and I am falling really, really fast. In my first fall semester, I didn't do so well in all aspects: social, grades, connections. I felt like I failed two times by spring semester because I got a lower GPA. My summer wasn't even going well, and now I have no classes, and school starts in 2 weeks. Honestly, I thought I wasn't going to see winter. I was, like, this is it. I'm not going to try as much. I can tell myself there's going be [a] tomorrow. I think that I was getting really tired of telling myself that there's going to be a tomorrow. When is it going to be the best tomorrow? So, it was getting a lot to handle. I was having those thoughts. It was just really hard.

The students' suicidal thoughts included physical exertion and fatalistic deliberations. Physical symptoms included headaches, loss of appetite, and fatigue. Several students talked about not having the motivation to get out of bed or to leave the home. On a psychological level, the mind was overwhelmed with consuming thoughts of death. Evelyn described their body as it experienced a panic attack while the mind considered the different passages to death:

> Usually, when I go through this part when I'm having a panic attack, I'll also have constant thoughts running and racing through my head. They often circle back: Oh, I want to die. I don't want to be alive. Sometimes, it would end up with me hurting myself. From day to day, sometimes I'd have passing thoughts of "I just don't want to be here anymore. I wish a car would come hit me. I wish I would develop cancer, so I had a reason to die." I was constantly looking for a reason to die.

In addition to considering death by cancer or a car accident, some students explored other methods of dying to alleviate their psychological pain. Some talked about taking the steps to remove a knife from the kitchen or putting a rope around their necks. Others spoke about their suicide attempts in more vague terms. Jamie talked about their suicidal thoughts and how that thought process led to an actual suicide attempt:

> I have consistently thought about crashing my car when I was driving. I've looked at how many pills it would take to overdose. I thought about what I would write in my letter when I would go. I've thought about jumping off a bridge a million times. I had every intention of doing it until it came to actually doing it. Something that would help me would be writing letters to people. I find that

more meaningful instead of writing a suicide letter to them. I would just write a thank-you letter because it would give me some type of clarity that I do mean something to someone else other than my sister. One time, I took a few pills, and it just made me sick. I stopped halfway through because I didn't want to do it anymore. I think that was probably the worst time and the closest time I ever got to doing it.

Jamie reflectively talked about the finality of suicide with these concluding thoughts: "I always felt like there was something worth being here for because once you do it, it's over. I was always just curious that maybe there's something out there that's worth living for."

This process of finding hope and promise in the midst of profound psychological challenges was a constant struggle. Students did not know when these thoughts or feelings would occur, and it made them vulnerable to triggers during inconvenient times. In general, it was never a convenient time to experience vulnerability; however, vulnerabilities were more manageable in the home environment than anywhere else. Thus, when triggers occurred, the goal was to make it home. Kelly talked about finding safety in staying home; however, when they were not at home and the suicidal feelings were pronounced, they wondered if they could make it safely home:

Some days, I really just wanted to stay home. Some days, I definitely reached out to friends or supervisors and just said, "I am not coming." I'm going to stay home and stay in bed to process those thoughts. I knew that driving a car when you are potentially suicidal is not the best idea. I've had certain moments driving home where I actually experienced anxiety attacks and panic attacks. It is very scary, and that, in turn, just kind of puts me in a very bad path, and it leads me more towards suicidal ideation. Incidences like that are scary because I'm just trying to go home, and I still feel this very negative energy. Coming to terms with those thoughts was definitely difficult, but it is something that helps me empathize with others who have gone through a similar experience.

When the participants did make it home to live through another day, there was a sense of relief, liberation, and sorrow. College students reflected on those who suffer from mental health challenges who do not make it home. On the one hand, they felt very fortunate to make it home safely; on the other hand, they are aware that many do not. Many felt the compassion and empathy expressed by Kelly, but they also explained the feelings of survivor's guilt. Cameron, a student who felt like dying since they were aged 10 years, discussed this prolonged reflection in a quiet and solemn manner:

It basically opened my eyes up to anyone really experiencing certain things that hurt this much. To be alive in general, it kind of helped me understand the fact that people are going through this on a day-to-day basis. Some are far worse than I am. Some have even, unfortunately, taken the actual steps of committing to killing themselves. I've had people around me who've actually done that. That's why it feels guilty for me to be alive. Sometimes, I think of this life as just something that I hated for so long that I wanted to be gone. But at the same time, there are others in my life who unfortunately couldn't even make it past as young adults even if they wanted to. I feel like . . . I think it's called the survivor's guilt. That impacts me a lot.

The participants shared their vulnerabilities in their compelling stories. The mental health struggles have been with them for years, and their expressions of pain in recalling feelings and thoughts mirror earlier works of suicide ideation among Asian American college students. In their weakest moments, they have lived to tell their stories and in the process looked to protective factors and developed an emerging resiliency to suicide deaths.

CHAPTER 2

# THE PROTECTIVE FACTORS AGAINST SUICIDE DEATH

The Centers for Disease Control and Prevention provides current information on evidence-based suicide prevention strategies.[1] The main goal of suicide prevention is to focus on decreasing suicide risk factors and increasing suicide protective factors. The provided information is useful for individuals, social groups, and communities. The following are some of the broad topic strategies: strengthen economic supports, strengthen access to and delivery of suicide care, create protective environments, promote connectedness, teach coping and problem-solving skills, identify and support people at risk, and lessen harms and prevent future risk.[2] Protective factors may include social support, physical health, self-esteem, coping skills, sense of purpose, and healthy thinking.[3] In other words, these protective factors may be viewed as characteristics associated with a lower likelihood of negative outcomes or qualities that will reduce the impact of a risk factor. For example, individual protective factors may include a positive self-image, self-control, or social competence.[4]

Protective factors are circumstances that keep individuals safe from danger. The more protective factors an individual embodies

*Stories of Survival*. Amy Wong, Oxford University Press. © Oxford University Press 2023.
DOI: 10.1093/oso/9780197662397.003.0003

or possesses, the more they are able to reduce their risk, in this case, for suicide ideation. Protective factors balance out the risk factors and act as cushions to safeguard an individual from risk. Another way of thinking about protective factors is to consider them as a safety net. Protective factors can be viewed as preventive measures to suicide death. The question to ask is, How does a person who experiences suicide ideation not take the next step to suicidal tendencies and suicide death? In other words, what are the factors that might help prevent an individual from taking steps toward suicide death? The research findings show that participants in this study embodied several protective factors that allowed them to move forward in their lives. They articulated that these protective factors gave them the strength and resolve to live another day. These protective factors made them resilient to suicide death.

The participants made it clear that mental health struggles are more pressing on some days and not too much of a concern on other days. However, mental health challenges do not truly ever go away because some have been living with depression, hopelessness, and suicide ideation since as young as age 10 years. Some days were more challenging than others, and there were days when they were not able to leave their beds or even their homes. At best, all they can do is live with and manage their suicidal thoughts and tendencies by utilizing protective factors. As stated previously, protective factors are qualities that contribute to one's general well-being and allow a person to be resilient in the face of challenges. A person with several protective factors—such as healthy coping skills, strong support systems, and individual mindfulness practices—will be better equipped to overcome life's obstacles, including living through the global pandemic.

# The Global Pandemic

The student interviews for this study took place during the first and second year of the global pandemic. Although this research focused primarily on the suicide ideation and resiliency among Asian American college students before the pandemic, I did include a question about their experiences during the emerging and evolving pandemic. Therefore, this section addresses their continuing resolve and determination to stay safe, healthy, and alive during the global pandemic.

Young people were already experiencing an increase in mental health issues before the pandemic. A Centers for Disease Control and Prevention report released in 2019 showed that the suicide rate among those aged 10–24 years increased 56% between 2007 and 2017. The rates of depression have also escalated, and there is an overall concern this generation is at serious risk for prolonged and enduring mental health problems. In addition, the stressors and trauma associated with the coronavirus pandemic are inflicting a greater psychological toll on young people. A survey focusing on the mental health of 18- to 24-year old adults in late June 2020 reported that 25.5% contemplated self-harm in the 30 days before completing the survey and 62.9% reported experiencing symptoms of anxiety and depression.[5] The global pandemic further aggravated existing mental health difficulties and struggles. A director for counseling and psychological services at a public 4-year university on the West Coast explained the negative impact of the global pandemic on college students: "Shelter-at-home orders have definitely led to students feeling disconnected and lonely. And those with problematic family situations may also face trauma or challenging dynamics at home, which can exacerbate existing mental health concerns."[6]

In addition to experiencing social isolation and challenging family dynamics, college students also faced learning difficulties, financial strain, and career uncertainty. Some students may have also tested positive for the virus and needed time to recover and heal from this potentially deadly disease. They may have also witnessed family and friends contract the virus and its devastating impact on their physical and mental health. Furthermore, some college students may have experienced the loss of a loved one to COVID-19. A director of the student wellness program at a 4-year public university on the East Coast noted that students also faced a high degree of "ambiguous loss." Ambiguous losses are considered less tangible losses, such as missing graduation or the final season on a sports team.[7] Students were mourning the loss of their previous life before the pandemic.

The global pandemic negatively affected the United States and deeply impacted the college students. Participants spoke about the abrupt changes to their academic and social life, including moving back to their family home, adapting to a new schedule, and adjusting to remote learning. They felt overwhelmed during the transition of moving back home and getting reacclimated to their studies in virtual spaces. They expressed feelings of anxiousness. Their stress levels were extremely high. Some had difficulty remembering specific events because "it was all a blur." The students articulated that things were happening very quickly because they were forced to abruptly leave campus. They were in constant motion as if they were on a never-ending carousel ride. During this period of constant change, there was also great uncertainty and fear about the COVID-19 virus. Students tried to remain current with the news while feeling nervous about trying to stay healthy. Participants recalled the early months of learning about the development of the global pandemic as a time of tremendous stress and exhaustion. It was a daily challenge to stay healthy and adapt to living with new requirements, including social distancing and mask mandates. Physical health was a main concern as they tried not to contract the coronavirus. Like many people throughout the world, these students were trying to stay alive.

As the college students transitioned back to their home environments, they expressed concerns for the health of their parents. They did not want their parents to die. Evelyn found that staying in the house was one way of keeping their mother safe: "I mostly just stay in because, again, my mom's chronically ill. But she just received the vaccine so we're all hoping we get vaccinated." Living at home during the first year of the pandemic was difficult for students because they had to adjust to their parents' schedule and worry about the coronavirus. Yet, there was the general concern for their parents' health and how they were going to live and survive together as a family. There were conversations about leaving the house for work or to grocery shop. These conversations extended to discussions about virus test sites and whether or not a person would be vulnerable to contracting the virus. The specific context generated stress and conflicts between parents and the college students. There was a general fear about the outside world once a person left the house. The parents and children were sometimes at odds with daily living as they adjusted to new information about the evolving pandemic. Keeping the lines of communication open and staying in contact with each family member was a useful survival strategy. The following is Taylor's experience about living at home during the first year of the pandemic:

I guess the most anxiety I get is from the idea that my parents still go to work and leave the house. It was extremely scary because I was able to take a leave for my hospital internship—that way I could stay home and not put anyone at risk, but then it's a matter of my dad still having to go to work because there's no way out of that. Then there's also that factor of them being scared to get tested and going to places that could potentially be the place where you could get infected. So I guess coping with those type of things and being able to sit down and talk to my parents without arguing. That has definitely been the most challenging but also the most effective way of getting to them. It's just talking to them and sharing information. I think now we're at a better place because they are also scared. That way it's easier to keep them at home, but no matter what there's always some incidents where you have to go out like you have to buy groceries. And it's just not that we don't trust them—it's more like you can't trust the next person outside. I guess constant communication with my parents and my family members has been the best way of coping with the pandemic itself. Yes, and just knowing what the next steps are until then.

Similarly, Dana expressed concern for their older parents because conflicts developed due to different schedules and habits. The transition of living at home with parents with different ways of living in the pandemic meant that students had to negotiate these generational dynamics. On the one hand, they wanted to be respectful of their parents' wishes. On the other hand, they needed to consider their own needs and well-being. Dana found that they could live in their family's home under their rules but still have an outlet for their much-needed social connections:

I think that it was harder over the summer since I was living at home with my parents. They're on the older side and they're super COVID conscious and I want to respect that but at the same time I'm 19 years old and it's summer and I want to go out with my

96

friends and everything. So that was kind of a source of conflict between my parents and I and also within myself. Moving down for the school year since I had a few in-person classes and I think that definitely helped and just being in a different environment is really nice. Also my sister moved to a nearby city for her job at the beginning of the end of the summer. So, sometimes I'll just drive up on a Sunday and spend the day with my sister. I like that it makes me feel more connected to people who I don't get to see all the time.

Students were focused on their own sense of well-being while also ensuring that they supported the processes needed for their parents' physical health. In general, staying healthy, clean, and safe were major themes expressed by the participants as they lived through the pandemic. For Dana, the social connections were crucial to their overall sense of well-being. Others found that learning about how to stay healthy and sharing that information with others contributed to their own safety and protection. Because new information was coming out regularly with changing rules, recommendations, and protocols, staying informed and current was a survival strategy for many students. Hayden talked about the importance of individual and social action by contributing to information sharing and enhancing the overall health of the world:

> For the last year, I would always share or repost any post on masks or any information about COVID or the vaccine when it was still in progress before distribution of it. I would keep a social distance and just stay in the house as much as possible. I don't think I've gone out with a friend at all. . . . At first, I liked wearing gloves but I stopped because it got a bit expensive to buy new gloves or to find them whenever we go to the hospital.

Participants discussed the importance of cleanliness as they learned more about the coronavirus. They viewed the coronavirus as unclean and unhealthy. Staying as clean as possible was considered as one measure to resist the spread of the coronavirus. They found that living in the time of COVID required more attention to staying hygienic and sanitary. Alex stated that staying personally clean helped during this time because "I like being sanitized." In addition, returning home meant students had to prepare and clean their living and study spaces. Jamie reiterated this point of individual and surrounding cleanliness: "Keeping myself and my environment clean is one of my main things because it stresses me out when it's dirty. It makes me feel like my life is a mess when my room isn't clean or my room is dirty."

This rapid adjustment was a challenge for many students, and even a year after the pandemic began, they were not able to fully acclimate to this new social order. In part, the rules were changing frequently, and it was not always easy to make adjustments. Students discussed how they were doing the best they could with what they had. In time, they learned that they might need to make life adjustments as new information came out about the pandemic. Some participants found that there was still great uncertainty in their daily lives. When asked about strategies they used during the COVID-19 pandemic, Quinn stated,

> I don't think I found the answer to this myself, to be honest. I feel just accepting that it's a part of our reality. Knowing that the COVID vaccine is going to become our yearly flu shot. I think, just acceptance and moving on.

In part, acceptance required staying current with the national news and campus information. There was an abundance of news and information about the global pandemic coming out each day. In fact, participants stated that all the news and information they were receiving was about the pandemic. There were many moments when they just felt overwhelmed with the pandemic information. Yet, they also believed that it was their responsibility to stay informed about the current events. Thus, students found it challenging to stay informed but not become overwhelmed with the news during this time of great social change. Taylor discussed the challenge of receiving information without being overburdened by too much of it:

> I think the biggest strategy was limiting how much time I was on my electronics and on social media. I think during break that was the most time that I had to really indulge in social media, and it was not helping me. It was conflicting between how much I wanted to be aware of everything that's happening and being up to date, but also how much do I really need to know without making myself feel guilty for not being able to do anything about it? I would say the most impactful thing that helped me cope with everything was not being so obsessed.

The initial lack of human interaction with friends was difficult for college students; therefore, they made the extra effort to communicate with friends and remain in touch. Individuals whom they used to see on a regular basis were no longer there in person. Students expressed that during this period of adjustment, their friends were the one thing that kept them going. Therefore, they made every effort to stay in touch. Shannon found that living through the pandemic was possible because of friends: "I'm continuously talking to my friends. Talking with my friends was kind of key to living under COVID." They explained that it was important to continue to stay in communication with the people they saw every day before they were required to leave the college campus. Kelly emphasized that the intentional social connection with friends required planning; however, it was important for friends to check up with and take care of each other from a distance:

> Something I started when we were in virtual classes was making a point to schedule one-on-one calls and trying to salvage some of that social connection that you get being in person. Everyone had to shift everything to a virtual platform. That includes your social hangouts. To just catch up with one another and assess each other's attitudes and well-being. I found that being able to schedule weekly calls or even daily calls with friends really helped me to finish as a student. Without those kind of moments, I feel like virtual learning does get very lonely. Making an effort to have some sense of social interaction beyond whoever you live with was really helpful for me.

Time was a theme among the participants. Students expressed that they had more time during the transition to remote learning because they did not need to drive to campus or walk to classes. They used this time to promote their own physical health. Approximately half of the participants indicated they used their extra time to engage in more physical activity, including playing basketball, practicing yoga, and working out. One student found that engaging in more physical activity had individual as well as family benefits. Morgan, an Xbox enthusiast, explained that taking walks was a good form of exercise because they stayed in shape while spending time with the family:

> I do a lot of walking. It was super easy to walk back home because we would have to take my dog out anyways. Back home during that five-month quarantine, my parents and my dog, and my grandma were walking. I was getting anywhere from 10,000 to 12,000 steps just about every day. I was in really good shape because we would go on a little walk in the morning. We would go on a four-mile walk

every night after dinner. We would eat dinner around 6:30 and walk at 7:30 or 8 and be home by 9:30.

Staying healthy and busy was a survival strategy for the college students. They used this time to stay safe, healthy, and well. In other words, they used this time to evolve, persist, and develop into stronger and more creative individuals. One student talked about using this extra time to spend outdoors and learn a new sport. Evelyn explained that learning how to skateboard had therapeutic and functional benefits while also helping them develop a new, enjoyable skill:

> I got a skateboard for Christmas. I've always wanted to learn how to skateboard. I know how to surf, but I'm very bad at skateboarding. I've fallen quite a few times, but it's fun. I had a lot of ankle injuries in the past, so I feel like it's helping with stabilizing my ankles. I just kind of hope that I get good enough so that it could be a mode of transportation because I hate driving.

Finding hobbies and learning new skills during the global pandemic was beneficial for the students. These new activities were healthy for their sense of physical and mental well-being. During the pandemic, students were even more mindful about adhering to a schedule. For example, they already had a routine or schedule on campus before the pandemic, and they learned that it was even more important to have a schedule at home during the pandemic. Several students highlighted the importance of maintaining a daily schedule or routine. Hayden said that "keeping that schedule I think I mentioned earlier, trying to maintain a schedule for yourself that way you give yourself a sense of normalcy." It was an adjustment period, and it took time to find a new routine, a new way of living through the global pandemic. Jamie discussed the importance of a routine to persist in their future goals: "Getting myself into a routine definitely helps because it's really easy to fall out of routine during COVID. Focusing on my professional career really helps my mental health because I feel instead of watching I'm actually doing something for myself." For others, focusing on academic and professional goals was not the most important agenda. Their focus was more on rest, relaxation, and family time. For Morgan, this routine focused on summer relaxation:

> Over quarantine it was the same routine especially when it hit summer because I was collecting unemployment. I didn't have to work. I was getting free money and I would get 8 to 9 hours of sleep, wake up and have lunch with my sisters. I would be doing whatever they were doing. My parents would be working and I would just hang out for 5 hours and then everyone would come home and we would have dinner. We'd walk. I'd watch TV with my dad or go up to bed and watch TV by myself. And that was my day for probably like two and a half to three months straight. It was great. I loved it. I loved being lazy and basically being paid to be lazy.

Overall, most of the participants adjusted to this new schedule and living in the family home; Cameron, however, did not do well during this time period. Cameron talked about how they have learned to manage their mental health struggles for many years; however, the coronavirus continued to add to their existing stress because they also had to worry about keeping their friends healthy and staying alive. Earlier psychological challenges became more difficult with the threat of contracting the disease. They also found that the usual coping mechanisms before the pandemic were not as effective in the COVID era:

To be completely honest, I don't think I'm managing it very well. I think it's very high stress, very, very, very high stress. About coping strategies, it's no different from what I would typically do. Just talk to my friends or listen to music. But the stakes are a lot higher because it's not just my life in danger. It's more so the people that I care about and the older people that I care about that are especially in danger. That puts very high stress on not just me but for anyone involved around me. If you told me, "How are you managing things?" I can't really give you a definitive answer. It's more about keeping my emotions in control so that I don't go crazy.

In contrast, Robin was coping well during the pandemic. They also indicated they were happier and thriving under these home orders and restrictions:

I was making myself a schedule. There will be two days of the week that I will allow myself to go to the grocery market with my mom and dad. I feel like it's getting better. Before COVID, my mom and dad work a lot, so we didn't see each other a lot, but because of COVID my mom stays home a lot, and my brother and my sister stay home. It makes me feel like my family is back together again. Before COVID, my brother and sister go to school, my mother will go work, and my dad will go to work. After school, when I come home, there is no one in my home, so it made me lonely, but now everyone is home every day. I am enjoying this time very much.

## Coping Strategies and Self-Reliance

Coping mechanisms help develop individual resiliency during times of psychological distress. The process of coping has been described as having willpower, self-control, as well as an endorsed belief in the ability to independently solve emotional distress.[8]

These are purposeful behaviors that individuals use when they are experiencing the challenges of daily living. It is taking responsibility for their own actions and behaviors to manage these mental health struggles. Although individuals may be experiencing a tremendous amount of psychological stress, they must learn to use their minds to reframe or reset how they address their problems. The individual cultivates their self-reliance over a period of time. The development of self-reliance includes the perspective "that even in the midst of an emotional crisis, an individual must be resilient and self-directed above and beyond what has already been endured."[9(p504)] Active coping includes using these behavioral or psychological techniques to reduce or overcome stress and pain. Active coping is intentional action that has been linked to psychological resilience.[10]

College students were intentional and mindful about using their coping strategies during times of great struggle. For many of the participants, learning to manage their depression and/or suicide ideation was a daily work-in-progress practice. Each day presented challenges and opportunities to work through their personal struggles. Many found the strength in their own abilities and determination. Although they acknowledged that they may live with mental health challenges for the rest of their lives, they were also strong-minded in working through their difficulties and struggles. These students learned to manage their mental health struggles by identifying the thoughts and actions that helped them in the past. They developed these psychological management skills by finding the processes and practices that helped them diminish their suffering and pain. For the college students, learning how to handle their mental health struggles on their own was a powerful indication of their determination and resilience.

Coping strategies involved individual activities. It was a daily challenge to live through the experiences with thwarted belongingness and perceived burdensomeness. Eleven participants expressed former or current suicidal thoughts and tendencies. Although Taylor indicated no suicide ideation, there were still visible feelings of depression and hopelessness. They talked about their experiences with burnout that came from the accumulated experiences of dropping grades, an overcommitment to student activities, and the lack of a healthy outlet to release the stress. Most participants experienced suicidal thoughts that highlighted deep sadness and loneliness. When asked what strategies they used to deal with sadness or loneliness, Evelyn responded, "I'm still working on those." All participants talked about coping with daily psychological struggles as a continuous process. It is a daily process to address their sadness or loneliness because some strategies worked in some situations but not in others. Some college students found pleasure and enjoyment in listening to music. Some listened to sad songs, whereas others preferred more happy songs. Students found pleasure and joy through the power of music in several different forms. Some described listening to music as their saving grace because music improved their moods and made them feel better about their lives. Listening to music was a simple and peaceful act. For example, Cameron found that an effective way for them to cope with stress was "to just go watch the sunset while listening to music." The joy of music was incorporated into their daily lives. Similarly, Kelly explained that music allowed them to move forward with the agenda for the day:

I still use music in my life whenever I feel that I need a moment to reset or simply just transition from one headspace to the next.

> I take what I call a music minute. I take either a song that's roughly a
> minute or a full song and just sit or lie down and really take in what
> that song means to me. Taking the lyrics or the melodies and really
> just immerse myself in that one song. And it takes no more than
> five minutes, and after that time is done, I feel more refreshed and
> ready to move on to my next agenda item.

In addition to listening to music, some students found contentment in calm activities such as reading fiction, spiritual, or self-
help books. Participants enjoyed the ease of reading and learning
something new in the process. They enjoyed being transported to
a new environment and relating to characters when reading fiction. The spiritual books offered ways to consider the meaning of
their lives, and the self-help readings provided them with tools and
resources to better themselves. Another soothing and relaxing
individual activity was writing in a journal. In these spaces,
individuals were able to express their feelings and emotions. They
were able to explore their thoughts in a quiet and reflective manner.
Journal writing helped them release their personal insecurities
and struggles. Taylor found that writing in a journal was an effective way to cope with sadness or loneliness: "I think writing out my
thoughts have been the most beneficial because it definitely feels
different from saying it out loud and then reading it." Thus, the
process of writing allowed students to consider their feelings and
work out their problems in a new way. Although it helped to talk
with their friends about personal concerns, participants found the
value of self-reflection that comes with journaling. The process
of taking a pencil to paper was also useful to organize the many
thoughts entering through their minds; writing by hand was a way
to slow down their thoughts. Dana used journaling to organize
and release their many negative and troubling thoughts:

I'll just write down a bunch of my thoughts in a journal. I do that because when I sense myself start to kind of spiral down, it's usually because I have a lot of thoughts in my head, and I just need to get them out.

In addition to journal writing, the power of reflection and release was also found in daily prayers. One student talked about sharing their feelings about difficult and challenging times through prayer. They found that it was not always useful to share their feelings and emotions with friends because they wanted to be considerate of the friendship; they did not want to overburden their friends. However, sometimes journal writing was not an effective way for them process their feelings and thoughts because they needed to be able to talk to someone. They wanted to talk with someone and use their voice to express their despair. As a result, they learned to enjoy spending time with themselves in prayer and reflection. Shannon stated the productive process of reflection and release:

Praying. I think praying is a huge thing. What I like to do is pray in my car or as I'm walking to class. I know that I was talking about spending time with people as a coping mechanism but I also like spending time by myself. I think that was a huge thing I noticed because I realized that when I don't—if I keep it all inside I might lash out at someone I care about. And so—sometimes I would just take time for myself and let the stress in before I destress with someone else. That's a huge thing I'm starting to learn—how I can vent and not take someone's energy with just venting.

One research study found that religious affiliation is a protective factor and may reduce the risk for suicide ideation among Asian American college students.[11]

Some individuals found enjoyment and pleasure in creative projects. Artistic endeavors allowed them to create a product with their own hands. They discussed how they made something useful and cool for loved ones and themselves. For example, Evelyn experienced joy in crocheting: "I've made a top for myself. I made a hat for my dog. I'm working on a hat for myself and a top for my friend." In this case, the gratification came from working artistically and making a product that will keep a loved one warm. These creative projects were satisfying and substantial for the students because they were able to share their creative talents with loved ones. Some students found happiness when making music. Cameron talked about their passion for playing the guitar for hours at a time. If they had any free time in the day, it would be spent on the guitar. During our interview, they showed me their guitar and explained that they usually kept their guitar nearby. These creative outlets had a calming effect on the participants, and it was a constructive way to turn the negative energy into more positive energy.

In addition to these creative outlets, participants used physical activity to manage their psychological distress. Students expressed the importance of physical activity and how it was a daily goal to stay physically fit and healthy. The act of moving their bodies helped release many forms of stress. These activities included taking walks, yoga, and running. Many of these activities were performed outside. Spending time with nature had healing properties for the participants. They enjoyed breathing fresh air and moving their bodies to stay active and healthy. Some did not choose one specific activity but, rather, performed a combination of physical activities to stay physically and mentally healthy. Exercise was important for most of the participants, and they found time in their busy schedules to fit in a workout. Alex found a productive combination of running and yoga to help relieve their stress:

> I like being active. I like running in the morning because it really clears my mind. It just sets my mind for the day and gets me going. I've also, in the past 2 years, 3 years, started doing yoga, and that has really changed my life for the better.

Student were very disciplined with their workouts. Even with a regimented schedule of classes and work, they made sure to include workouts as part of their daily activities. Whereas several enjoyed the great outdoors, others found more structure and comfort at the gym. The indoor gym offered various exercise machines so the participants were able to work out in a variety of different ways. Students explained that physical activity was necessary because of the daily academic pressures and stress. Getting daily exercise was a high priority for college students. For Shannon, the gym was a stress reliever to address their overall physical fitness:

> One of the major big factors that kept me going was a gym. I was very disciplined in that aspect. I always made time for the gym, whether it be after class at night or, like, the 30 minutes before my next class. I always make time for it. The gym was definitely a nice coping mechanism.

After a long day of classes, winding down was something to look forward to. The rhythm of moving their bodies was refreshing. Some participants indicated that their physical exercise came from walking to and from classes. They enjoyed this time of being outside and experiencing the healing benefits of being surrounded by nature. Students spent a lot of time walking around campus and walking to and from classes. They used this travel time as part of their healing time. For example, taking a different path to and from home and exploring new spaces was particularly meaningful for participants. The simple act of walking from one location to another was an enjoyable and refreshing activity. Getting outside and walking was an intentional activity that they looked forward to at the end of the day. For Robin, the quiet act of walking and spending time alone was comforting and relaxing:

> I will try to go out of my house more. For example, after the class ends, I will not go straight to my home. I will enjoy myself by walking around campus or study in the library, or just find a coffee shop and sit there to refresh my day.

The time spent alone in nature had healing properties.

Relying on their own skills was important to their overall sense of well-being. Their coping strategies were not static, and students found that they needed to be flexible to changes. What may have worked in one year may not be as productive in another year. Something that was effective yesterday may not be quite as effective today. For example, as people entered and exited students' lives, the students eliminated some coping strategies and added new ones. One student talked about changing coping strategies over the years. Hayden discussed their earlier solitary activities and how the coping strategies now included more social interaction with loved ones:

> This is where my coping strategy of just diving into social media or YouTube or any streaming service started. Since I had no one to go to, I just let myself enjoy whatever I'm going to be watching. For all these years, it's been helpful. But now that I have a girlfriend who understands me, I can talk to her sometimes, or at least she lets me release my emotions. I think there have been times I put

unnecessary baggage on her because I've been alone for so long. Since I'm not used to making long-term friend commitments. I think of my sister, who is 13 now. We sort of relate more, and we have more of a connection than when she was just a kid. I discuss things with her, and that really helps me out.

Acceptance was also a coping mechanism. College students explained that sometimes doing nothing was also an option because there were some emotions and feelings they could not change. They explained that sometimes they just had to accept these current feelings and live with them. They learned to reflect upon these experiences with the hope that there are better days ahead. Participants lived through these rough moments in a day by reflecting on the events. Part of self-reliance was adjusting their mindset to accept the current challenges with the hope that the future would be better. It was the acceptance that most people will have bad days but that these bad days will not be repeated. This mindset helped college students manage the current crisis with a more hopeful perspective. Shannon talked about this mindset with a focus on the future:

> I think what got me through those days was—I guess at the time it was hard for me to realize this but now I'm a little bit more in touch with my emotions. I'm realizing that what got me through those days was realizing that there's always tomorrow. If something bad happened I'm like okay well I don't have to repeat today. What always got me through is telling myself that today will never happen again. This specific day will never come again, so what could possibly go wrong?

Individual coping mechanisms involve focusing on the present situation. Research on mindfulness has examined suicide ideation. *Mindfulness* is defined as the process of paying attention to present-moment experiences with acceptance and nonjudgment.[12] The research team outlined that mindfulness may be a significant factor for suicide resilience because it focuses on how one reacts to and copes with stressors. Moreover, the research team established that mindfulness may act as a strategic and adaptive process to cope with adversity effectively, such that these negative circumstances do not diminish the perception of and attachment to a life worth living.[13] Therefore, coping strategies are intentional behaviors that assist students in living with more meaning and purpose in their lives. Although individual coping strategies were productive for students, they also found the need for support systems.

## Support Systems and Human Attachment

American psychologist Abraham Maslow outlined basic human needs in a pyramid called the hierarchy of needs, a theory of psychological health centered on fulfilling basic human needs. One important psychological need is belongingness, which must include intimate relationships and friends.[14] Human beings want to experience a sense of belonging in their families and communities. It is from these private and social spaces that individuals experience love and companionship. To be with others, then, is to be human. In order to thrive and survive, human beings need other human beings. In other words, human beings need social support. The research shows that social support is considered a protective factor against suicidal behavior and suicide deaths. The presence of social support and the behavior of seeking social support have been associated with psychological hardiness and flourishing in the face of major adverse life events.[15] Accordingly, individuals need the love, support, and sense of belonging that come from other people.

Participants discussed protective factors in the form of support systems. Many students talked about the meaning and importance of friendships. They talked about their long-term friendships that began in elementary school or middle school. There was also a discussion about more recent friendships from high school and college that included classmates and roommates. Several participants identified emerging and important friendships with members of a fraternity or sorority. One study found that being a member of a fraternity or sorority was a protective factor.[16] In addition to peers, participants also listed faculty members, mentors, and counselors as members of their support system. Students recognized that each person of their support system may serve a different need or purpose to them. There were conversations they had with roommates that they would not have with a faculty member, and there were conversations they might have with a mentor that they would not have with a childhood friend. College students valued the diverse support members in their life because they explained that they were not meant to experience life alone. Cameron called these individuals that made up their support team a true blessing:

> I can't do this alone. Thankfully, I'm very gifted with the amount of people in my life. I think I tell myself every day that I am the luckiest person alive because I've had these resources. I've had these people to bring me back up from where I once was, and they don't expect anything out of it. I think the whole counting your blessings thing is a very viable option to really rejuvenate your thoughts and get the ball flowing of positivity.

Participants had much to say about their family members. Although the family was a source of pressure and stress, it also provided strength and security. This duality of the family unit was not easy for participants to talk about because it was difficult to reconcile their feelings of appreciation and disdain for their family members, particularly their parents. However, for many, the feelings were more clear, and they looked to the family unit as a source of love, support, and strength. In the family unit, there were many family members to count as a source of support, especially when it included extended family members. Without hesitation, Morgan talked about their immediate and extended family as being the core of their support system:

> I would definitely say my immediate family, like my parents and my sisters, but then you also have all of my mom's immediate family. My mom is one of six siblings, so, I mean, all my aunts and uncles. I'm the oldest of 13 cousins, so all the cousins and my grandparents.

Whereas some college students talked about the support they received from various and specific family members, others discussed the limitations of parental support. Students recognized the financial support they received from the parents, including shelter, food, and clothing. They conveyed deep appreciation for having a place to live, food to eat, and clothes to wear; they were aware that they were more fortunate than other people. However, they also expressed disappointment with the lack of emotional support from their parents. They expressed frustration and impatience because they were not able to openly and authentically talk with their parents about their feelings and emotions. Participants have made the effort to share their struggles with their parents, but they found that their parents were disinterested in their experiences. In some situations, the students believed there were misunderstandings when they tried to have a conversation with their parents, and both sides left the discussion feeling unsatisfied. Students believed that their parents were uncomfortable is this type of personal sharing from their children. Over a period of time, these conversation voids resulted in a general acceptance of lesser communication between parents and children. Alex accepts that they cannot have a meaningful conversation with their parents; therefore, they seek love and support from their friends:

> My parents don't really know how to deal with emotions very well. So, I don't really go to them for that. I've tried before, like, calling my mom or dad, but that doesn't really get anywhere. I get more emotional help from my friends.

On the one hand, participants did feel a connection with their parents because their parents raised them and provided a home for them. On the other hand, they believed that although this connection was familiar, it was not close or intimate. Participants described it as an important—yet distant—relationship. The relationship that students had with their parents was important to them because it provided them with the foundation to live their lives. The students desired a bit more from their parents. Although their parents were not emotionally available, participants empowered themselves by seeking more productive social supports. Kelly explained that although they are close to their parents, there may be cultural practices that do not generate an emotional closeness to their parents that they have with close friends. When asked who they count as members of their support system, Kelly replied without hesitation:

Definitely friends. I don't know if this is the same for other Asian American college students or just other people in general, but I tend to share more about my struggles with my friends than I do with my family. I don't know if that's a cultural thing or not, but it's something that I observed within myself. So peers and very close friends make up the core of my support system. Beyond that, it is my family, of course. I do live with them, and we are very close. I'm very fortunate, but I don't go in depth or detail with my family as I do with my friends.

Several other college students reiterated the general unease of talking with their parents about emotional concerns; however, they looked to other family members for emotional support. In this manner, many still found a strong support within the family unit. Furthermore, students found that the presence of their parents in their lives was enough; they did not need to have de-tailed and extended conversations with them because just having them in their lives was important. Although participants did not feel comfortable talking freely with their parents, they did find it easier to talk to specific siblings. In part, students felt a more emotional connection to their siblings because they were of the same generation. Some students reached out to older siblings, whereas other reached out to younger ones. Taylor found that sharing information with their siblings was helpful because they were close in age:

> I would definitely count my siblings and a select few friends. I would say they all support me in very different ways. It's not always easy to talk to my parents about anything, but just knowing and having reassurance that they're there for me has really helped. Through the years, my siblings have literally been through everything with me. I don't think I could ever be as bare-bones as I am with them with anyone else. And then, with my friends, just having a sense

of community that we are the same age. I don't really know a lot of people the same age that really understand what I'm feeling or give me the sense of comfort that some of my friends do.

The role of parents was discussed by several participants, and many acknowledged that although it was reassuring to know that parents were present, they were not always emotionally available. Students explained that they felt a physical security knowing their parents were around in the home, but they felt emotionally safer with their siblings when it came to sharing their insecurities and challenges. In some situations, students talked about not feeling physically safe because there was physical abuse at home. Participants acknowledged that among their friends, physical beatings were common knowledge, and they did not want to address it further in our interviews. Instead, they focused on the good relationships in their home. While some participants did not feel physically safe around their parents, they did feel emotionally safe with their younger siblings. Evelyn looked to their younger sister for emotional support and comfort:

> I know that my sister likes to call herself my therapist even though she's not qualified at all. She's my younger sister, but she likes to listen to me talk about how I'm feeling, and she checks up on me. I know both my parents are there but are kind of emotionally unavailable because of the childhood trauma they went through. My mom's Korean, and it's kind of known that they beat their kids and whatnot. Same with my dad.

Several participants discussed their support systems with the rule of three. The three main members in their support systems included friends, family, and therapists. This was a running theme in that it was not one person who was their sole supporter; instead, participants talked about having several important people in their life. For example, Robin talked about the different roles that are played in each of these relationships, including other college students, a younger sister, and mental health specialist. Robin was able to exchange information with other students about common struggles with being first-generation college students. In this manner, this student was able to understand that they were not alone in their struggles. In the relationship that Robin had with their younger sister, it was more about being a good role model or taking care of this younger sibling. They also enjoyed spending time playing with their younger sister. Finally, learning to open up to a counselor was a new experience, and these conversations are still emerging and evolving. Robin found a support system with all three groups and discussed these three different and useful relationships:

> Usually, I will talk with my friends a lot because we came all from the same background: first-generation students to go to college. When I came here, they were also new to the U.S. as well so we get connected and talk to each other and share our stories. I also play with my little sister. She's younger than me, so she has a lot of energy. I'm also starting to talk to the counselor, and I am starting to open myself more.

The rule of three important members in a support system was also explained by another college student, Dana. The best friend from back home provided a historical foundation for this college student who felt that they could always rely on their best friend even if they were geographically far away. At the same time, this student also found support and comfort with their current roommates. Although these were new and emerging relationships, they were also important because they were physically nearby; thus, there was immediate social support, if needed. Finally, it was instrumental to have a large group of people from whom one could find support and community. For Dana, their three support groups included a best friend, roommates, and their sorority:

> I had an assignment asking who I would go to if I needed help. I listed my best friend from back home. She's in another city right now, which is tough because we can't see each other. Even though I know she's busy, I text her all my feelings, and I know she'll get back to me later. My roommates are definitely part of my support system because they're usually always around. They know me well enough, so they can talk me through stuff that I need help with. Finally, I have my sorority. I know that if I need somebody to open up to, they are understanding. They always make a safe space for any of the members to open up and be vulnerable without judging them or making them feel bad.

Participants talked about the emotional support they received from specific family members and close friends. These supportive individuals shared activities with the vulnerable college students, including eating meals, watching a movie, going to the beach, and having conversations. Whereas some individuals talked about the importance of family and friends in their personal lives, others discussed the importance of having professional support. In these situations, they looked to members of the college community for life experience advice. Kelly identified faculty, advisors, and mentors as leaders they looked to for words of wisdom or insight. Shannon valued her family members, significant other, and best friend; however, they also needed the professional support that came with supervisors and other colleagues:

Personally, it would be my family. My siblings, I'm very close to them. My parents, they are always supporting me. And my partner, who I've known since high school. Being with someone who's also on the same road as me is really comforting. My best friend is such a great person that I don't even have to explain something to him. He'll just know, and he'll know how to comfort me. Those are my personal support system, but then I also have professional support because sometimes my family might not know how to support me professionally. Professionally, it would be my supervisor. She is so different from my last supervisor. I'm still trying to get used to appreciating the different style she has being my supervisor.

Sometimes, there was one person who stood out for college students. One person made all the difference in the world. Although they may have a small community of friends, several students identified one person in particular for encouraging them to go on when things were very difficult. It was the one person who made all the difference in helping them honor their humanity. It was that one friend who kept them alive. For Cameron, it was a specific person and a specific group of people who helped with their overall survival:

One of my best friends. She's been there since I was 17 when the whole thing happened. I think she's been a very big impact as to why I'm still here. I think people like her, as well as this little friend group that I still have and cherish to this day, showed me that showing love and empathy and those emotions don't make you vulnerable. They make you human. Previously, I was very sheltered in that aspect. I was very scared of showing empathy, showing vulnerability to other people. I feel that is a very big crucial part in understanding certain mental illnesses like anxiety. I think that without her, I probably wouldn't be here today.

## Life Skills and Self-Care

Life skills are learned over time, and they help ensure human survival. Self-care has many aspects, but the focus is on the individual. It is the care that one provides for their physical and psychological well-being on a daily basis; it is taking care of and healing the body and the mind. Life skills are developed over time, and several participants stated that they were still in the process of learning what worked best for them, particularly when the global pandemic impacted their studies and they needed to test out new life skills. Self-care is also mindful activity that enhances the quality of a person's life. Life skills are essential to human development and survival. Life skills include basic activities such as managing nutrition, sleep, money, possessions, and time. Individuals are encouraged to take more responsibility for self-care and self-management as they grow up.[17] In addition, self-care practices are activities that maintain and promote physical and emotional health and include healthy eating, sleeping, exercising, and socializing behaviors. Self-care practices accentuate the positive aspects of health and well-being.[18]

All participants had a daily practice of self-care to promote healthy living. Two college students each described three activities that they performed to meet their specific day-to-day needs. For example, Taylor summarized their daily self-care goals with this statement: "Eating my meals. Cleaning my room. Playing with my dog." Kelly also indicated specific everyday practices as a form of self-care: "Eat, sleep, and hydrate." Students listed the most important activities that they tapped into when they considered taking care of themselves. Because many were away from their parents, they needed to also promote self-care skills as they lived more independently from their parents. This was due in part to living on campus and was also a product of becoming adults. The skills they developed when they lived with their parents continued to serve them well as more independent college students. One way to develop life and survival skills is to live with intentionality. For example, a study on college students' mental challenges found that making the time for personal wellness and lifestyle habits increased commitment to self-care.[19] Self-care included taking care of the body and mind. Self-care practice was a return to basic daily needs. Dana described these human needs as follows:

> I feel like I have to go back to the basics. I want to shower every day. I want to try to eat three meals. Eating has been kind of a struggle sometimes. I do try to set goals for myself and to do things I enjoy. If I'm eating dinner, I might watch a show that I enjoy. I definitely like music. If I'm going through something and I need to calm myself down, I like to listen to music. A while ago, I was doing yoga and stretching in the morning, which was actually really nice. I just need to work on keeping up with it and not being lazy. Other self-care stuff, face masks, and putting on makeup to feel better about myself, to feel more confident about myself. It makes me better in general.

Daily living includes routines. College students anticipated these routines as part of their daily living. Research has highlighted the importance of creating and following a schedule so that individuals are not overwhelmed with options and choices:

> Having clear routines can cut down on the overwhelming choices we tend to face on a daily basis and can also lead to less uncertainty.

In an otherwise stressful time, it's important to build up those routines, even if we have to make arbitrary ones ourselves.[20]

The importance of a routine or schedule was a major theme for students as they talked about how they took care of themselves.

The routines involved healthy practices that helped individuals take care of their bodies. Participants viewed following a routine as a form of self-care, as Jamie explained: "I consider my routine as a form of self-care. I keep myself in check like having my morning cup of coffee." This form of self-care began at the start of the day, paving the way for a more productive day. Having a little bit of caffeine in the morning helped the mind and body wake up, and it helped set the tone for the day's activities and events, as Jamie continued with their thoughts:

> Sometimes I try to read in the morning when I'm up for it. And that is probably the best activity for self-care because it helps clear my mind a little bit more. So my self-care in terms of my wash days is just so when I don't feel so good about myself on the inside in my head, then it makes me feel better about my outside appearance, the way my body feels instead of the way I feel about myself as a person.

Others described their daily routine with a specific concentration on practicing good hygiene. Several college students talked about the important of taking care of the body. They understood that it required time and energy, but it was a necessary activity that positively contributed to their overall well-being. Taking care of their bodies kept them healthy and gave them the self-confidence to confront the day. Some college students talked about the specific parts of the body to which they gave more attention. For example,

Hayden stated, "Every Thursday I cut my nails just to make sure I'm keeping myself together." Other body care focused on the entire body. This included taking care of the inside and outside of their bodies. In general, taking care of the body was of great concern to the college students. Morgan talked about their day with detailed activities that focused on taking care of their body and keeping it clean, healthy, and rested:

> I'm very diligent with my hygiene. I brush my teeth, and then I floss my teeth, and then I use mouthwash. I wash my face twice a day, shower once. I do like the brushing and flossing and mouthwash. I wash my face when I wake up in the morning, and when I go to bed, I'll shower. At some point, I'll shower after I go to the gym, but if I know that I'm not going to go to the gym that day, then I'll shower in the morning. I try and get anywhere from 6 to 7½ hours of sleep, eat two meals a day. I really only eat lunch and dinner.

Morgan's diligence also applied to the sleeping hours. Morgan was very specific about how the hours were spent in rest and activity. They did not use more time than was absolutely needed to attain full rest. When I mentioned that 6 hours appeared like a limited time for a full night's sleep, Morgan replied:

> It's rare that it is 6 now. It was 6 probably more during freshman year just because it was hard and people living in the dorms there's always someone to talk to. I would say now I try to get at least 7. I kind of work my way backwards and think, oh, if I need to wake up at this time, what time can I go to bed? For example, I needed to wake up this morning at 8:50 a.m. so I told myself in order to get 7 hours of sleep I needed to go to bed at 1:50 a.m., but I really ended up going to bed at 1:15 a.m. I mean, it's mostly at least 7 hours. On a good day, I'll hit 8 but I sometimes find it a lot harder to get up when I get more than 8 hours of sleep—I feel like I'm oversleeping.

Each hour was important for the college students. Time was valuable, and they were specific about how they used their time. To stay on task, students set their phones to remind them of specific daily tasks. Even if they performed the same tasks each day, it was helpful for them to have daily reminders. For example, Evelyn stated,

> I have a reminder list. So I get a reminder in the morning to brush my teeth, a reminder at night to brush my teeth, a reminder to take my medicine. And then at night, I try to do this skin care routine every day.

In addition, individuals discussed taking care of their bodies as an expression and extension of self-love. The research on self-love includes the themes of mindfulness and compassion. One study focused on college students and mindfulness. Students were encouraged to monitor their daily physical activities and to examine their eating habits as practices of mindfulness.[21] Mindfulness is connected to compassion skills. Collective mindfulness and compassion include the conscious regulation of attention; awareness of self (body and mind); awareness of others; attitudes of openness, empathic curiosity, and trust; and care for self and others. In other words, enhanced mindfulness predicts increased self-compassion.[22]

Several participants highlighted the specific practice of a skin care routine because it was an enjoyable process that made them feel better about themselves. Taking care of their skin made them feel more beautiful and loved; they also enjoyed the time touching their skin and nurturing it with special creams and lotions. Taking care of their skin was a solitary act and they enjoyed it immensely.

They appreciated the time with themselves as they used assorted soaps and lotions. Taking care of their skin was a form of self-affirmation. As described by Robin, the time they spent taking care of their skin increased the love they felt for themselves:

> I'm starting to use skin care. It's a process. I enjoy the process, and it makes me feel like I love myself more. Every morning when I wake up, I go to the bathroom and look in the mirror and talk to myself and say, "You will get through this. Everything will be okay." These are the strategies I have to enjoy myself.

Focusing on one intentional activity was a form of self-care. This allows for paying attention to the details of the chosen activity. It allows the participant to center their focus on the one event. Paying attention is being present in the moment and being mindful of intentions. The research on intentional activity encourages individuals to stay focused on one task:

> We're all used to multitasking, especially when watching lectures or videos on our screens, but data suggests that doing so is cognitively exhausting and can impact our mood. In fact, research shows that we feel better when we're being mindful than we do when we're mind-wandering to other tasks. Commit to single-tasking—put your phone away if studying or watching lectures on a laptop, commit to a specific time period when you're "at school" versus doing other leisure activities or texting with friends.[23]

Several college students highlighted the importance of physical activity as a form of self-care. As previously mentioned, students talked about physical exercise as an individual coping strategy during stressful and distressful times. They explained that physical activity allowed them to release negative thoughts and feelings in a productive way. In this context, students expressed physical activity as a form of self-care. One student stated, "I like doing something active every day." College students enjoyed different forms of physical activities, including going to the gym, playing basketball, and practicing yoga. Taking care of their bodies was a form of self-care that was also beneficial to the mind and spirit. The goal was to keep moving and stay active. One important goal was to make sure they did not lay in bed all day; rather, it was productive to recognize that body movement was good for the body and the mind. Quinn explained it as follows:

> I feel like when I lay in bed all day and not moving your body is just scientifically proven to not be healthy. I know that I've said yoga to a lot of things, but I recently started that during the first semester when things were happening. Yoga is the one big thing that definitely got me out of that. It releases endorphins and yoga has a meditative aspect to it, too. I get some time to do some positive self-reflecting instead of wallowing in self-pity. I get to think about things I'm grateful for—my gratitude—so that's been really good for me.

Exercising was a mood changer. Exercise made people happier, and it was a way of taking care of the self. Practicing self-care is important for human survival. Shannon proudly stated that "going to the gym is like self-care for me." Working out made the college students feel happy, and they found great pleasure in gaining better skills in their particular sport. They discussed that repetitive physical activity was good practice for developing athletic skills. Sometimes, they engaged in their sport like a professional athlete. Hayden stated, "I work out or try to do physical activity as much as possible whether it's lifting weights or my favorite just playing basketball. Just imagining that you're your favorite NBA player and making a buzzer beater."

The most important self-care routine involved food and eating. Most of the participants talked specifically about food and eating as a form of self-care; this included shopping for groceries, preparing meals, and eating meals alone or with others. Eating healthy foods was a source of good mental and physical health. Alex stated, "I like cooking and preparing my own meals and going grocery shopping. I learned that when I put good things in my body, I feel better mentally. I just feel better overall." For the participants, eating was not just a necessity for survival, it was also a process of enjoyment and pleasure. There was also the goal of working toward a healthier diet, and several college students stated that this was a work-in-progress journey. Daily eating was connected to staying healthy. Cameron talked about the physical aspects of eating and self-care: "Recently, I've been eating healthier in terms of tracking what I'm eating, tracking the calories, tracking the exercise, stuff like that." Similarly, Hayden appreciated the physical comfort of eating food: "I eat a lot. I just like feeling full in my stomach." Furthermore, Shannon discussed eating with purpose: "Eating good is a way of taking care of myself. I'm a lot more intentional with what goes on my plate." The goal of a healthier diet involved being selective about the foods they ate. For many, there was true joy in preparing meals for themselves, some of which were based on family recipes. When they prepared foods using family recipes, they also felt a connection to their roots. Alex found enjoyment and comfort in one of their mother's recipes:

I like cooking and preparing my own meals and going grocery shopping. I learned that when I put good things in my body, I feel better mentally. I just feel better overall. I learned the easiest kind of comforting food I can make is fried rice. I use my mom's recipe. She taught me, so I do that a lot, and it's one of my favorite things to eat for dinner.

Whereas Alex ate this meal alone while in college, some noted the simple pleasure of eating with other family members. College students enjoyed the communal act of spending time with family members through the activity of cooking at home. It was something family members could do together, or it was an act that one person could perform for other members of the family. Thus, cooking with or for family members was a way of sharing with or giving to loved ones. Family recipes were celebrated, and it was a way of bringing family together as a form of self-care. During the global pandemic, more students spent time at home with their families. Kelly described the comfort and joy of cooking a specific dish for the entire family:

> I find a lot of joy in cooking. Because we went to virtual learning, I was home more, and I was able to cook more. In my time as a virtual student, I think cooking as a form of self-care is underrated. It definitely allows me to connect with my heritage and cook more Asian foods. There's a Filipino dish called sinigang. It's like a soup or stew usually made with pork or beef and various vegetables. It's something that brings so much joy to my family. I tend to make it, especially in winter. I make it every couple of weeks because it helps me through the winter months where it might be colder, and I might feel more lonely, or I have various trauma related to the winter months. Cooking this dish brings me a lot of joy and respite from thinking about all the negative things.

Table 2.1 shows sample statements regarding the participants' self-care routines.

Table 2.1 Participant Responses to the Interview Question: What Are Some of the Ways You Take Care of Yourself Every Day?

| Participant | Sample Statement for Their Self-Care Routine |
| --- | --- |
| Alex | "I'll light a candle every now and then. It helps." |
| Cameron | "I've been really getting into skincare." |
| Dana | "I kind of have to go back to the basics . . . to shower, to eat . . ." |
| Evelyn | "I have a reminder list to brush my teeth in the morning and at night." |
| Hayden | "Every Thursday I cut my nails just to make sure I'm keeping myself together." |
| Jamie | "I just keep myself in check like having my morning cup of coffee." |
| Kelly | "Eat, sleep, and hydrate—so really addressing basic needs." |
| Morgan | "I'm very diligent with my hygiene." |
| Quinn | "Yoga has a meditative aspect to it. I get to do some positive self-reflecting." |
| Robin | "I'm starting to use skincare. I enjoy the process and it makes me feel like I love myself more." |
| Shannon | "Going to the gym. I've taken up journaling." |
| Taylor | "Eating my meals. Cleaning my room. Playing with my dog." |

## "Today Is a Good Day"

Having a good day is an example of a positive life event. However, there is not much research on the impact of positive life events as a protective factor against suicide ideation, suicidal behaviors, or suicide deaths.[24] In the current study, the future was an important topic for college students because they were working toward it. However, they were also mindful of the present. In the same way that bad days had a prolonged negative impact on a person, good days had a prolonged positive impact. The moments in a good day allowed students to find happiness in the present. These good moments had a sustaining positive influence on the individual's well-being for the whole day. The accumulation of good days helped college students work through some of their more challenging issues because they believed in the possibility of better days. They knew there would be better days to come because they experienced good days in the past. Students were asked what accounted for a good day.

College students revealed the special moments in a good day. While they shared stories about daily college challenges, the participants also enjoyed the pleasures and joys of a good day on campus. Proper rest the night before made for the beginning of a good day. Evelyn stated, "A really big part of having a good day is getting a good night's sleep. Making sure my body is fine. So, making sure I eat something, making sure I'm alert and awake." Feeling rested allowed students to be more productive in their day. For Quinn, a good day is "any day where at the end of the day, I feel productive like I did something good whether that's with school or just for myself like exercise." Almost all the participants talked about preparing for the next day with a planned schedule. For example, scheduled weekly activities with friends gave students something to look forward to. Taylor explained this important time with their friends:

I used to have weekly lunches with some friends, so those helped me to look forward to later in the week. Just knowing that at least whatever happens from the morning 'til then I'll still have that moment with that friend. I think in terms of friends and lunches, it's nice because we're all so busy and knowing that there's a dedicated time that I'm giving to someone, and they are giving to me. Just being with other people that want to be there with me and to just spend time together. I think that's pretty important.

Some participants looked forward to special days in the week. These special days included scheduled activities or usual routines. They talked about looking forward to these days because they were meaningful to them in some way. These days included a planned activity or the opportunity to spend time with friends or a special person. Some participants talked about specific days in the week as anticipated good days. Evelyn looked forward to Fridays:

I was a cheerleader for my first 2 years in college. So, Friday mornings, I'd have practice, which leaves me feeling energized because I'm working out all those endorphins. Then, I take a shower, go to class, and then I'd meet up with friends, maybe go out, and that would be a really good day for me. So, usually Fridays.

For Dana, an anticipated good day fell on a Monday:

My freshman year first semester, on Mondays, I had classes with my friend pretty much every single class. We had classes from 9 a.m. until about 8:30 p.m. We had every single class together, and we would go to the lecture halls and then Starbucks. We studied together between classes. We'd walk together. It was just fun to always have somebody to talk with. I'd say that's probably one of the best overall memories that I have.

In addition to having weekly special events or anticipating special days spent with close friends, planning was the key to a good day. They found that because they were very busy, having a schedule helped them organize their priorities and get things done. Several students elaborated on the importance of maintaining a daily or weekly schedule. For example, Hayden explained how good planning was one factor to accomplishing goals:

> From what I've learned about myself over these last 3 years in college, I'm a third-year, I feel really accomplished when I've done a lot of activities or that I've completed a bunch of homework assignments or I did some chores that I wanted to do or things that I've been putting off and finally completing them. I think it's being achievement-based. I think that's the term. I also like it when I have a schedule for myself. I find that to be really helpful during this quarantine time, so getting all these achievements done all within this schedule that I've set up for myself, that's a really good day.

Getting up early to focus on the day's activities was meaningful for the college students. When asked what was most important for having a good day, Alex discussed waking up early: "I think getting up early in the morning; I feel like I need that every day." Participants enjoyed starting their day early in part because they had a busy schedule. In addition, they highlighted the need to maintain a routine and keep a schedule. The schedule was their guide for the day. Morgan further discussed the importance of getting up early, was specific about how each hour would be spent in a day, and described this structured day as a good day:

> I would say a good day for me is waking up anytime between probably 8 to 10 a.m. I will get my homework done, maybe squeeze in a workout or two in the morning. Probably eat lunch between 11:30 to 12:30, but only spending about 30 minutes actually eating while watching a show or a movie. Maybe attend my classes and have everything wrapped up by 4. I'd say 2 hours working on homework after that because I try and get all my work done before dinner, so

I can just kind of chill. By 6:30, I will either cook something or go out with my roommates or my sister, who is a freshman here. We'll get something on her meal plan, which has been very nice, followed by coming back in and hanging out with my friends and probably finishing the night off with 2 or 3 hours of Xbox.

Several students talked about the classroom experience as setting the overall tone of a good day. They reiterated that they were in college to learn and to receive an education, with the end goal of earning a bachelor's degree in their chosen discipline. They further highlighted that their main purpose was to earn a degree so that they could be more competitive in the workforce. Thus, classroom learning was a major part of their daily schedule. Taylor described a good day as follows: "A good day on campus before COVID was going to class and understanding what I was learning." Similarly, Shannon learned by absorbing the information from a classroom lecture:

> I think, honestly, a good day for me is when I know that the professor will make space for just listening. I think I feel like my day starts to get anxious when I feel like I'm in a space that I have to ask questions. Sometimes, I just like to listen and really get into it so a good day is when the class is just to listen. Let me take in the lecture.

In contrast, Cameron appreciated lighter classroom days: "As a college student, I guess no class might be a pretty good day. It might be a pretty good one with no work. No undesired work is a good day."

In addition to good academic days, college students also found enjoyment in the company of their friends. The path to earning a degree was not just about studying; it was also about cultivating friendships that could last a lifetime. Companionship was important for college students, and they articulated the need for friends in college. They appreciated the time they could spend with their friends, even if it was just a few minutes a day. When asked about the highlight of their good day, Jamie stated, "I would say the small interactions with my friends on campus." Moreover, Robin enjoyed their breaks because it was a time when friends from different campuses could gather in their hometown to be together. Kelly enjoyed the security of being in a protected safe space with friends: "Being able to be in a community space where I could freely express my identities and just to feel very welcome and safe and have the ability to be authentic within that space made for a really good day." The accumulation of good days contributed to one of their main reasons for living.

## Reasons for Living

Mindfulness includes reflecting on the meaning of life. Researchers have noted that depressed students experienced personal insights that allowed them to find meaning in their lives. These students found that going to school, earning their degrees, and gaining a better financial future were purposes for living.[25] The meaning of life can be broadly defined as a sense of purpose that is believed to matter in a way beyond the individual living that life; in addition, the meaning of life construct may be a coping mechanism to buffer suicide ideation.[26] The researchers surveyed 585 undergraduate students, of whom 19% were Asian American, and found that the presence of meaning in life partially mediated the relationship between perceived burdensomeness and suicide ideation and fully mediated the relationship between thwarted belongingness and suicide ideation. Thus, individuals who were able to find meaning in life were able to better cope with emotional distress and mental challenges.[27]

In a 2015 study of suicidal Asian American college students, researchers collected data about their purposes for living. The sample comprised 58 Asian American college students from 70 different universities and colleges.[28] In their own words, students made the following statements:[29]

> My desire to do something meaningful with life.
>
> Suicide will only end the beginning of my life. There's still a great deal of something out there for me. I look forward to finishing school to gain a better future.
>
> There was a small voice in the back of my head that told me I was giving up before I started. And giving up is such a pity. I felt I hadn't given back anything to the world, and I wanted to do that before I died. That more than anything, restrained me.
>
> I was born in a third world communist country. People who are there will give anything to have what I have. I must be grateful of the things that I do have. . . . I should be grateful to have that chance to experience anything.

In another study, researchers found five factors that informed Asian American college students' reason for living: survival and coping beliefs, college- and future-related concerns, responsibility to friends and family, moral objections, and fear of suicide.[30]

In the current study, all participants articulated reasons for living. Each person found the motivation to live. They found the motivation to survive even when they experienced deep and disturbing thoughts and emotions. They explained that although they experienced challenging days and that there were moments when they did not want to live, there was always a small part of them that still wanted to go on. It was not always easy to get to the point of moving on, but they generally soldiered on. There was a part of them that wanted to lived. The desire to live came from finding a purpose to keep going. They found purpose in something or someone to keep them going every day. Participants discussed the challenges of daily life, but they also found determination in their friends, family, and the future. Participants also talked about the importance of individual responsibility and taking charge of their own lives. Jamie stated the importance of doing the work themself because what keeps them going was "myself because no one can do it for me. That's the only thing that can really keep me going." For the students, the belief in the self also included the knowledge that they were needed by other people around them, including friends and family members. They understood that they had the ability to be present and available for themselves and other loved ones, both people and pets. Quinn stated what kept them going: "My friends are definitely number one for me. My dog." Evelyn maintained a mantra that kept them going each day and was a daily reminder of their responsibility to other people:

> Something my friend said to me while I was not well. She said, "You need to be here." Anytime I'm kind of feeling like I don't want to be here, I'll remind myself that I need to be here. I need to be here for my friends, for my family. That's all I need to do. I don't need to become a doctor. I don't need to do all these things. I have my health. I just need to be here. So, that's what's really been keeping me going, just repeating that to myself.

Shannon reiterated the need to be here: "I like giving back to my family. I think that that keeps me going because I haven't been able to give half of what they've given me, so that keeps me going."

In addition to giving back to their family, they also considered their obligations to people they have not met yet. They thought about the people they would come into contact with in the future. This was a powerful incentive to carry on because it showed that participants had a future orientation:

> I think what keeps me going every day despite how hard it was in college was the kind of life I envisioned for myself. The group of people I'd like to positively impact. What keeps me going is that there are people out there I haven't met yet who, when the stars align, I need to be there.

Participants also found the incentive to persist because the family was a source of their inspiration. There was joy in their voices when they spoke about their beloved younger siblings. They demonstrated their passion and purpose when talking about their younger loved ones. They wanted to be role models to their younger siblings; they wanted to set a good example for them to follow. Some had a very deep connection to their younger siblings, who they loved very much. Robin equated hope and promise with their younger sister:

> It's my little sister because she's 5 and I'm 22, so there is a big gap of age. I saw the process of my mom delivering her, so it makes me feel very connected to her. I feel some responsibility toward her. I want to give her everything that I have. She gives me the will to go to the end of my day.

Participants also talked about the gratitude they felt for their parents. They understood that they were fortunate to have a good life because their parents provided them with the opportunity to become successful. In these moments of reflection, college students honored their parents by recognizing the benefits and resources they received from them. In many ways, these students viewed their parents as role models and wanted to follow their example. The family was a source of inspiration. Morgan talked about reproducing the family success as their source of motivation and persistence:

> The thought of being able to provide and succeed the same way that my parents have. I want to succeed for them. I want to be on my deathbed knowing that I did everything I wanted. To be on my deathbed knowing that I was fluent in Spanish, knowing that I served 30-plus years as a firefighter, knowing that I was able to provide for my kids while also living a financially healthy lifestyle, similar to what my parents are doing right now.

In addition to important people in their lives, participants believed in the promise of the future. Although many expressed uncertainty and ambiguity about the future, they also believed that the future would bring better days. To the college students, the future was about hope, promise, and possibilities. The desire to work through the challenging days with the belief that things would get better was a powerful incentive for them to keep going. Participants talked about the past, present, and future; they believed that time was on their side. Hayden proclaimed that the present is better than the past and that the future would be even better than the present:

> I'm an optimistic person. I'm well aware that today is better than 1 year ago, 5 years ago, 10 years ago, 100 years ago. I've always known that, so I've always gotten confused when people say, "Oh, my God, today is worse than ever before." I'm thinking, "No, it's

not." No way. We are so much better than what we were before because we're human, we're people, we learn, and we evolve. We make things better for our future selves or future generations. I've always understood that without anyone having taught it to me. I feel like that's always been my thing that kept me going: I know things will get better.

The promise of the future made the present bearable. Participants articulated their hopes for the future. Even if the future was an unknown entity and the days seemed to drag on, there was always the desire to see what the future had in store for them. They also believed that the future had to be better than the present. Cameron stated, "The hopes of me accomplishing my goals and dreams. As long as I have that, I think I can keep going, at least for now." They believed that the current bad days would be counterbalanced by the future good days. They believed in the possibilities of the future. The students articulated their ideas about the balance of the world. They explained that good days and bad days were a part of life. They did not expect every day to be a good day, but they also believed that not every day was bad. Good and bad days were just a part of life and people will experience a range of emotions and feelings in a lifetime. Kelly explained that the balance of a human journey was a combination of the dark days and the bright days:

> I think just being able to appreciate life and the complex range of emotions that we have as human beings. Something that keeps me going is knowing that, yes, I might have a really bad day, and I might feel very negative. I'm leaning into my depressive tendencies, and I might just not have any energy. I know there's always a way out, and there's always a counter emotion and opposite emotion. There's that opportunity to feel joy and happiness and fulfillment.

Even when I'm in those dark moments, there is a sense of privilege
to feel that range of human emotion.

One emotion communicated by the participants was compassion for others. In their suffering, they still wanted to be in service
of other people. In part, their own suffering gave them a care perspective for others. They viewed the world through the lens of
compassion. Although they were also in pain, they knew that they
would accomplish their goals, some of which included helping
people. They wanted to make a contribution to other people who
were also suffering and needed help. They were working toward
a helping profession. Students were willing to work through the
temporary negative emotions because they wanted to be of service
to others in the future. Alex conveyed it as follows: "Knowing the
fact that I will be a nurse someday, that I will be successful. I'm
going to reach my goals. I know that there are just so many good
days ahead." For some, living through a global pandemic made
their work even more meaningful. This time period motivated
them to continue to work toward their future goals. The future
was a common theme among the students I interviewed. Taylor
also looked to the medical field as a way of helping others in the
future:

> The future. I think that having a goal really helped me get through
> everything. It is definitely present in my academics. Before COVID,
> I used to serve shifts at the hospital almost two times a week, and
> those were always on the weekends. Those shifts would get me
> through the week of classes. I know that these weekly shifts help
> until I get to a place where I can call this my career, so that's what
> gets me through because I enjoy doing that. Now with COVID,
> I want to allow myself to look forward to being in a situation where
> I could help others and do something that I enjoy. Yes, the future.

The future included realizing their goals, helping individuals, and giving back to their community. Participants believed in a better tomorrow for all people. This future orientation with them in it gave them the incentive to move in the direction of their goals. They knew that the path was not always smooth, but they believed that they could be of service to other people in the future. It was the future that they looked to; it was the future that kept them going even against all odds. Dana also wanted to work in the medical field and give back to their community:

> What keeps me going? Academically, what keeps me going is that I really want to help people in the future. It's something I know that I want to do, and it's motivating because even though lectures can get boring and I can get really tired, I think about all this stuff that I'm learning now is going to apply to my future. I'm going to be using this and helping people, so it makes me feel like there is an end goal in mind. It's not like I'm taking notes on this lecture for no reason.

Coursework was difficult, but participants believed the difficult work would help prepare them for the future. Although each day was a challenge, they truly believed that they would succeed and reach their goals in the future. For many, it was monitoring one day at a time. They knew that if they could get through one day, they could get through another. They used this process as a way of moving forward. The participants had a forward-motion perspective. They just kept going. Making it to the end of the day was a meaningful goal for the students. Dana further explained that they had to make it through each day to arrive at a better future:

> All I need to do is get to the end of the day. I know that's not the best, but sometimes that's all I can really do. When I'm feeling hopeless,

Table 2.2  Participant Responses to the Interview Question: What Keeps You Going Every Day?

| Participant | Sample Statement for What Keeps Them Going Each Day |
| --- | --- |
| Alex | "I will reach my goals. There are so many good days ahead." |
| Cameron | "The hopes of me accomplishing my goals and dreams." |
| Dana | "All I need to do is get to the end of the day." |
| Evelyn | "I need to be here for my friends, for my family." |
| Hayden | "I know things will get better." |
| Jamie | "Myself. No one can do this for me." |
| Kelly | "Being able to appreciate life." |
| Morgan | "The thought of being able to succeed like my parents." |
| Quinn | "My friends are definitely number one for me." |
| Robin | "My little sister. I want to give her everything that I have." |
| Shannon | "The kind of life I envisioned for myself, giving back to my family." |
| Taylor | "The future. Yes, the future." |

something that gets me through is I just have to tell myself: It will get better. Reflecting on past times where I felt the same way and think about how I got past that and just seeing that I did it once and that I can do it again. I will do it again.

Table 2.2 presents sample statements of what keeps the participants going each day.

# CHAPTER 3

# ADDRESSING THE PARADOX OF SUICIDE VULNERABILITY AND RESILIENCY

Colleges and universities have been providing educational services to students for a long time, and that will not change in the near future. Generations of young adults have earned their degrees and moved on to careers, and there will be many generations of college students to follow in their footsteps. It is hoped that these individuals will find meaning and joy in their work lives as they use their training to make the world a better place in which to live. As these young people move into this path of productivity and independence, they learn to support and provide for themselves after receiving the necessary tools and resources to do so . However, while they are passing through the system of higher education, all stakeholders at the university level must also support and provide for the college students. In fact, college representatives who make a career as administrators, faculty, and staff are hired to provide a specific service to college students, the main stakeholders. Still, individual offices and departments do not do this alone. Systems of higher education do not carry the sole responsibility for the care and development of college students. This is a responsibility that the world shares by looking out for and

*Stories of Survival.* Amy Wong, Oxford University Press. © Oxford University Press 2023.
DOI: 10.1093/oso/9780197662397.003.0004

taking care of each other. In this light, college professionals will never replace parents, but there are compelling reasons to provide students with all the necessary tools and resources they need in order to academically succeed while on the college campus.

As students make their way to their chosen college campuses, it is hoped that they will enter a nurturing environment in which they will grow, develop, and learn. This new place will become their other home for the next few years, and they will be guided by a different set of responsible adult leaders. *In loco parentis* means in the place of the parent.[1] There is a historical practice in the United States of viewing university faculty as temporary substitute parents for students. For example, students who entered college before the 20th century did so immediately after eighth grade, and faculty served in loco parentis. During this time period, the faculty focused on student learning, character development, and the regulation of students' behavior. In general, the college environment was a large family unit in which individuals slept, ate, studied, and worshipped together. Faculty members were considered the parents, and students were considered the children. Throughout the years, students' rights on campus were expanded, and more personal responsibility was placed on the students. The notion that college representatives should serve a parental function for students has long been abandoned. Today, the expectation is that college students will regulate their own behavior, use their time effectively, complete assignments on time, and seek academic assistance as needed.[2] In addition to being held accountable for their academic progress, college students must also be responsible for managing their physical and psychological health.

Each year, new and returning students with mental health challenges arrive at college campuses to work on earning their undergraduate degrees. Among these students, Asian Americans aged 17–24 years are the group most vulnerable to hopelessness, depression, and suicide ideation.[3] In addition, Asian American college students reported higher levels of suicide ideation than European American college students.[4] Thus, Asian American college students will have additional struggles while working on their university degrees. A large part of the college experience for students is to interact with other members of the university community in residence halls, classrooms, and open campus spaces in order to generate a sense of collegial belonging while working on educational goals. However, experiencing psychological difficulties may become a barrier to a student's overall campus participation and academic achievement. The well-being of students has been a concern of university officials for years. Fulfilling the goal of supporting all students with varying needs against declining financial budgets has been a delicate balance for university administrators as they make decisions to eliminate or maintain certain student services. Furthermore, college students expect a certain amount of available psychological and counseling services as they work toward their educational and professional objectives. Therefore, there is a crisis in higher education as more students enter universities with mental health struggles and may need to rely on campus resources to achieve their personal, educational, and professional goals.

I interviewed Asian American college students who have experienced suicide ideation to learn how they used coping strategies, support systems, and life skills to develop suicide resiliency. They shared with me that they experienced risk factors that deeply impacted their suicide ideation. These risk factors exacerbated existing mental health challenges and difficulties. In other words, these risk factors made Asian American college students more vulnerable to suicide ideation. However, they also shared with me that they experienced protective factors that prevented suicide death. These protective factors mitigated existing mental health challenges and difficulties. In other words, these protective factors made Asian American college students resilient to suicide death.

Using a narrative practice, one-on-one interviews were conducted to understand the college students' experiences with suicide ideation and resiliency. The main goal was to listen to the stories of college students and to generate meaning from their lived experiences. The conversations were conducted during the global pandemic when college students were engaged in off-campus remote learning. Although several students expressed Zoom fatigue and exhaustion, they all wanted to share their stories with me. They wanted to be heard especially during this time period when the media gave more attention to the rise in anti-Asian language, confrontations, and violence in the United States. This was a moment in history that hearing and sharing their stories became even more important. This moment included their history with mental illness, living in a global pandemic, and seeing violence against Asians and Asian Americans. During this distressful and dangerous period, there was a greater sense of urgency for systems of higher education to gather evidence-based research to support Asian American college students.

## Understanding Vulnerability and Reducing Risk Factors

Theories of suicide framed Research Question 1 by focusing on Asian American college students and their experiences with suicide ideation: What is the experience of suicide ideation among Asian American college students?

Six major themes of distress and pain emerged in response to Research Question 1:

1. Students shared their history of mental health challenges.
2. Students articulated the continuing struggles that stem from their family's intergenerational trauma.
3. Students identified the difficulties that come from accumulated bad days.
4. Students explained they do not feel a sense of belonging on campus.
5. Students discussed their feelings of guilt when they believe they are a burden to other people.
6. Students described their current and ongoing suicidal thoughts and behaviors.

These themes of vulnerability are risk factors to suicide ideation.

## Theme 1: A History of Mental Health Struggles

The first theme focused on the history of earlier mental health challenges of the college students. They experienced hopelessness, depression, and suicide ideation during the middle school and high school years. These periods were particularly difficult for them because they did not know how to process their feeling and emotions. It was a time of confusion because they did not understanding their negative moods. Some faced more transitory suicidal thoughts, whereas others suffered through more prolonged suicidal thoughts.

The more fleeting suicidal feelings would come from an immediate conflict, such as having a heated argument with their parents, and would usually go away in a short period of time. On the other hand, the more prolonged suicidal inclinations lasted for years and continue to endure in the present day. Moreover, it is a continuous effort to manage their history of mental health challenges. When the students were younger, they were puzzled by their unstable temperament, but as they grew older they developed an acceptance of their continuing feelings and emotions. They arrived at the understanding that this was just who they were, and they learned to live with it.

In time, they experienced loneliness and isolation because they were not able to articulate their daily struggles with psychological distress. Sometimes, they were able to share their negative deliberations with a close friend, but they often found that some friends were not very good listeners. As a result, those sharing their feelings of suffering were made to feel like a burden to their friends; this further isolated the struggling students with feelings of loneliness. Other daily struggles, such as the academic pressures from their parents to earn good grades, further aggravated their sense of hopelessness and depression. The psychological agony was so overwhelming at times that some students thought about the different ways they could die by suicide. In their imagination, they considered jumping off a bridge, overdosing on sleeping pills, and intentionally getting hit by a car. Some have even composed suicide notes in their heads to loved ones. Several college students discussed seeing a counselor or therapist, whereas others did not mention if they were receiving mental health resources or support.

## Theme 2: Intergenerational Trauma

The second theme is the existence of intergenerational trauma within the family unit. Students stated that their parents have lived a life of suffering and misery. They speculated that their parents' difficult lives may have originated from their own abusive and violent family upbringing. For example, the students learned that their grandfathers experienced physical and psychological trauma when they fought in wars; at the same time, their grandmothers experienced extreme deprivation and hardship living in a war-torn country. Witnessing extreme suffering and violence on a massive scale left survivors of war in a damaged psychological condition. In other words, students explained that their grandparents had been diminished from war, and this negatively impacted the upbringing of the students' parents. Grandparents who lived through violence raised their children with aggression and cruelty. In turn, when these children grew up and became parents themselves, they used some of the same parenting methods on their own children. Thus, the students explained that the physical abuse and emotional neglect they received from their parents contributed to some of their own psychological distress. In this way, intergenerational trauma continues with each succeeding generation. Students have suggested that physical and psychological trauma not addressed in one generation would get passed on to the next generation with devastating consequences.

College students indicated that they grew up in a family environment in which their parents were emotionally unavailable. These students stated that they were not able to speak honestly about their negative emotions with their parents. Although some students tried to open up to their parents, others felt that their parents were not concerned with their moods and feelings as long as their children were housed, fed, and clothed. As long as they received the necessities in life, the parents were reassured that their children were doing well. Not having a close relationship with their parents was a disappointment for the students. They understood and accepted that their parents would not change their parenting styles. Although they accepted their relationship with their parents, they imagined a different kind of relationship with their future children. They believed it was possible and desirable to raise their own future children in a more openly loving and nurturing manner. This future was a long way from the present time; thus, students did not elaborate on the specific details of what this parenting style would look like. Moreover, although they did not indicate specific different parenting practices, they asserted that they will work very hard to not reproduce the examples set by their parents.

## Theme 3: An Accumulation of Bad Days

A description of the accumulation of troubled days was the basis of the third theme. A challenging moment or experience during the day could be overwhelming because it contributed to the overall heaviness of the already present college stress and academic pressures. Earning a college degree is a difficult journey; if it was an easy process, more people would hold university degrees. Difficult days in college do add up. The amassing of difficult days added up over time to weigh the students down. At times, this collection of demanding situations in a day was devastating for students because they expressed feeling inundated and exhausted with classes and course assignments. College students were very serious about their educational goals as they organized their daily activities in a planner. The purpose of each day was to stay on a schedule and complete each task; however, if they deviated too far from their daily agenda, it then became a never-ending cycle of falling behind and trying to catch up. Therefore, a daily goal was to stay on schedule so that they would not fall too far behind. Sometimes this was made particularly challenging when they also needed to address their mental health difficulties. In addition, having relationship problems with family members or close friends created anxious and tense reactions for students. They did not enjoy having arguments and conflicts with loved ones because they felt helpless about being able to achieve a more happy and peaceful relationship in the immediate future. These interpersonal quarrels also distracted them from their studies, thereby generating more pressure and stress in their daily lives. Although the college students understood that good days and bad days were a part of life, they highlighted these more rough circumstances to emphasize that an accumulation of daily challenges and struggles aggravated their overall mental health. A rough experience or a terrible day will be unpleasant and inconvenient for most people; however, rough patches in a day for a psychologically vulnerable person can be pronounced and shattering. Some students intentionally tried to maintain a positive outlook on life, but it was not easy to do after many years of experiencing psychological anguish and continuing disappointments.

## Theme 4: Thwarted Belongingness

The fourth major theme explored the emotional state of college students and their experiences with a lack of meaningful connectedness at their university. Students did not feel a strong sense of belonging on campus; most expressed the sentiment that they did not feel a sense of belonging on campus at all. Thwarted belongingness included struggles with cultural adjustments and social expectations, academic challenges and imposter syndrome, and racial tensions and campus racism. New college students faced a period of adjustment as they were introduced to the norms, expectations, and culture of campus life. There were new guidelines and rules to follow, and it was not always easy to know what to do or whom to ask for more information. This confusion and lack of direction only contributed to their sense of isolation. For students living on campus, learning to live with new people and taking academically challenging classes were sources of great excitement but also generated nervous feelings as students tried to make positive social connections.

On-campus students often felt anxious because they were far from home and knew they could not just go home when they encountered negative social experiences. In time, they learned to find safe and comfortable spaces for themselves as they focused on their studies. As they lived with a bit more ease on campus during the semester, they found that they had to renegotiate a sense of belonging when they returned home to their family environment during academic breaks. This back-and-forth journey between the home environment and the college campus created unease and anxiety for students as they reacclimated to reentering each residence over the years. On the one hand, they lost a sense of security when they left their family to begin a new life as an on-campus college student. On the other hand, they lost a sense of independence when they left their college campus to resume their former life as their parents' child. Thus, the college years were marked with cultural shifts and adjustments as they lived in different home environments.

Students who lived at home during the university years learned to develop new identities as commuter college students. Although their home environment did not change, they still needed to make the transition from high school graduate to new college student. For commuter and residential students, there were social expectations of participating in school activities and joining student organizations. After all, most wanted to have a fun and exciting college experience. However, they did not always encounter a welcoming environment in some student organizations and sometimes experienced feelings of rejection by their peers. These negative experiences made them feel sad and left behind; some students conveyed feelings of anger and resentment. In addition to these sentiments of not feeling socially accepted, students continued to feel the heavy weight of academic challenges, including scholastic competition, failing grades, and impostor syndrome. Students attributed their lack of belonging on campus to their underdeveloped scholarship; they believed they did not belong on a campus with people who were more intelligent and achieving academic excellence. In this manner, students expressed their deep-rooted academic insecurities and did not feel worthy of being college students.

Lack of belonging was also associated with witnessing racial tensions and experiencing campus racism. Students spoke about racial hostilities in the classroom, residence halls, and open campus spaces. They focused specifically on the model minority myth, racial microaggressions, institutional racism, the perpetual foreigner myth, and pandemic scapegoats. First, students explained there was the false perception by faculty members and student peers that they possessed natural superior academic abilities due to the prevailing model minority myth. This viewpoint meant that student peers believed that Asian American college students would be in a position to tutor them in various academic disciplines, and faculty members assumed Asian American college students did not require additional educational support. These repeated incorrect assumptions continued to perpetuate stereotypes about Asian American college students. These stereotypes further alienated and isolated Asian American college students from the campus community. In the interviews, students clarified that sometimes they were not doing academically well in a class and would benefit from additional educational support; however, they did not believe they could express these thoughts to student peers or faculty members because they felt they would not be taken seriously. These experiences contributed to their feelings of "otherness" and isolation. On the one hand, they were seen as intellectually superior and not comparable to other college students who were more academically average. In other words, they were deemed as a special type of college student. On the other hand, because they were seen as academically gifted, faculty members did not give them needed academic attention and they were often left alone to their own resources.

Second, students elaborated on their campus experiences with racial microaggressions. In the campus spaces and at student gatherings, students often felt invisible to those around them. When students navigated the campus spaces to travel from classroom to classroom, Asian American college students sometimes had to make room for other students to pass. There was the belief that in the limited physical spaces during class transition periods, Asian American college students were usually the ones to make the sacrifice to get out of the way or students would run into each other. They expressed that there was a sense of being ignored or unseen by other college students; this feeling of being invisible to others was a reminder that they did not feel a sense of belonging on the college campus. Furthermore, Asian American college students found that other students did not talk to them when they were in a small group of students involved in a robust conversation. They felt intentionally ignored because other students did not make eye contact with them and would only talk to people who were not Asian. In one incident, an Asian American college student stated that one person approached the group and purposely positioned his back to them in order to not see them at all. Asian American college students did not feel a sense of campus belonging when they were ignored and made to feel invisible.

Third, students articulated the lack of an Asian American Studies program at their college campus as an example of institutional racism. They described how this nonexistent major contributed to their feelings of not being important to the university community because there existed academic programs honoring other racial and ethnic groups, including Africans, African Americans, Latino/a, and Latinx populations. The students were upset that their university did not support promoting the presence and visibility of Asian Americans in the United States. The absence of an Asian American Studies major, minor, or program was profoundly felt by the students. In addition, the university community is not given the opportunity to learn more about the history and culture of Asian Americans in an academic environment. The lack of an Asian American Studies program is a form of muting or silencing the Asian American experience. This program policy may also be associated with the perception that Asian American college students are doing academically well and do not need the support of an Asian American Studies major or minor to reinforce a collective racial identity. For the students, the campus message is that there is no room or need for an Asian American Studies program or that this program does not belong at the university. In other words, it is a low institutional priority.

Fourth, Asian American college students provided examples of how they were made to feel like a foreigner on the college campus. They shared that their residential living situation was less than ideal because their non-Asian roommates made negative comments about their cultural practices. These disapproving remarks emphasized to Asian American college students that they were different from other college students; these differences were perceived as odd, strange, or unusual. Asian American college students had to explain why they took off their shoes when entering the living space and left them by the front door; they were criticized for the foods they ate because these were viewed as unfamiliar and smelly; and they received complaints about listening to Chinese music and were told to turn off the offending songs when their roommates came into the room.

The fourth point of being viewed as a perpetual foreigner in the United States is associated with the fifth—and final—point of being pandemic scapegoats. At the time of this writing, Asians and Asian Americans had become scapegoats for the developing global pandemic. In virtual spaces, they were belligerently accused of eating bat and aggressively blamed for the origin and spread of the coronavirus. During Zoom calls with members of their affinity group, they were infiltrated by non-Asians and attacked with racist names and hate-filled messages. The college students I talked with expressed their shock and anger when they were attacked in virtual spaces. Asian American college students were perceived as different or foreign to other college students; their perceived foreignness made it easier to blame them for the dangerous COVID-19 virus. Being made to feel like a perpetual outsider or foreigner is a constant reminder to Asian American college students that they are not valued members of the campus community.

## Theme 5: Perceived Burdensomeness

The perception of being a burden to others was the fifth major theme. These stories were directed at family tensions and financial concerns as well as friendship obligations and emotional overload. Participants described being a financial burden to their parents because they were taking too long to graduate or they were not performing at the academic level that was expected of them. The tremendous academic stress magnified when their parents constantly asked about their grades. For the students, schoolwork was time-consuming and difficult because it was a never-ending cycle of attending classes, working on assignments, and taking exams. Many felt the academic pressures of university work. In addition to working diligently in their classes, the students also conveyed the demanding expectations of trying to live up to other high-achieving members in their families. However, they did not always feel capable of accomplishing the same level of academic and professional success as their older siblings. The students wanted to make their family members proud and to know that their parents invested financially well in them. Instead, they sometimes felt blamed for spending their parents' money as perceived underachievers.

Students also found themselves worrying about their families while they were away at college. In addition, they felt like a burden when they thought their parents and other family members were feeling anxious about them while they were away at college. They did not feel good about themselves when they considered that family members would agonized about them. Feeling like a burden to their family members contributed to their overall sense of frustration and shame for using the family's limited resources of money, time, and energy. The students stated that feeling like a burden to their families made them feel worse about themselves. Sometimes they felt consumed by guilt and sadness. These heavy emotions of sadness and guilt contributed to more psychological pain.

Similarly, participants expressed deep concerns about overwhelming friends with their personal feelings and emotional struggles. Although they were willing to be emotionally available to their friends, they felt a profound sense of guilt if they put too much emotional responsibility on their friends. They stated that friendships involved mutual sharing; however, they were still working through feelings that they were equally deserving of the same love and compassion they extended to others. These thoughts placed a tremendous weight on the college students because they wanted to be able to share their feelings with friends, but they also believed that they were overburdening their friends with too much information. This sense of guilt further contributed to their emotional suffering. The college students wanted to be good friends to others by allowing them to talk about their suffering; however, they believed that being good friends also meant that they did not overshare and overextend with their friends.

## Theme 6: Ongoing Suicidal Thoughts

The sixth major theme offered descriptions of the students' ongoing suicidal thoughts and behaviors. Some college students experienced self-destructive thoughts and behaviors at a young age and these continued into adulthood. For others, these fatalistic thoughts and tendencies emerged in the middle school and high school years. A few believed these were usual feelings for young people and believed they would grow out of them. For most, these feelings were confusing and caused stress and anxiety because they could not be controlled. Negative emotions and feelings could arrive at unexpected moments and students gave attention to those emerging developments. In time, these repeated psychological disturbances became normal to them. As college students in the present time, they now have a better understanding of their mental health challenges. However, living with psychological difficulties is still a periodic challenge and struggle. Even though they have lived with their mental health struggles for years, it is still not easy. In fact, the experience is very weighty and demonstrates the power of accumulated struggles and difficulties. College students learned the different ways to live with depression and suicide ideation, but they explained that managing their mental health challenges remain a work-in-progress.

College students continued to confront ongoing suicidal thoughts and behaviors. They explained that their psychological distress was aggravated by burnout, academic failures, and financial hardship. Furthermore, suicidal thoughts sometimes followed panic and anxiety attacks. Students portrayed these feelings of helplessness and powerlessness similar to falling into a hole. It was a hole they could not get out of. In essence, they felt trapped and alone. They also shared their experiences of suicide ideation and described what they thought about to end their profound suffering and pain. Some of these mental visuals included wrapping a rope around the neck, overdosing on sleeping pills, jumping off a bridge, getting hit by a car, and cutting themselves with a kitchen knife. There were daily thoughts about death and thinking about ways to die as some considered leaving a suicide note thanking their loved ones for being in their lives. The thoughts sometimes led to action as they opened a bottle of medicine and stared at the pills. Thoughts of death were usually present as the students imagined the different ways to end their pain. When these suicidal thoughts passed, the students were grateful for another moment. However, there was always the concern that they would not make it to the end of the day or through another season.

## Understanding Resiliency and Promoting Protective Factors

Theories of resiliency framed Research Question 2 by focusing on Asian American college students and their suicide ideation management strategies: How do Asian American college students who experience suicide ideation use coping strategies, support systems, and life skills to work through suicidal tendencies during their time in college?

Six major themes of endurance and determination emerged from Research Question 2:

1. Persisting in the global pandemic
2. Utilizing coping strategies and self-reliance
3. Cultivating support systems and human attachment

4. Developing life skills and self-care
5. Celebrating the accumulation of good days
6. Remembering the reasons for living

These themes of resiliency are protective factors against suicide death.


## Theme 1: Persisting in the Global Pandemic

The first resiliency theme focused on persistence under the global pandemic conditions. I interviewed students in the first year of the global pandemic (fall 2020 to spring 2021), and I was moved by their resolve and determination to continue their studies and to develop coping skills in this period of great uncertainty and disruption. They voluntarily participated in our interviews, which indicated to me that they wanted to share their journey at this particular time in history. They were not deterred by another Zoom meeting. They wanted to share their experiences with me. Although there were many stories of difficulties, pain, and struggles, there was mostly a desire to be heard so that others may learn from their experiences. They wanted to let others know who suffer from suicidal tendencies that they are not alone. To me, this was a powerful indication of their tremendous compassion and resiliency.

During the transition from campus brick-and-mortar learning to off-campus remote learning, students abruptly acclimated to online classes at home. The students showed a strong sense of determination to continue with their studies in this new learning platform, although they spoke about the challenges of relying exclusively on their computers for their education. Perseverance was the key to successfully learning in virtual spaces. The lockdown further exacerbated their preexisting mental health challenges. The abrupt changes in their structured learning and forced isolation compounded their depression and anxiety. In addition to staying committed to their schoolwork, students also learned to develop their time management practices under these new and emerging circumstances. They learned to limit their technology time when they were not participating in classes, they attempted to remain in contact with a few classmates and close friends, and they made the effort to spend more meaningful time with their family members.

Students were also focused on keeping their parents safe and healthy during the pandemic period. They were mindful of limiting physical contact with others to keep the household clean and uncontaminated. Furthermore, the students concentrated on keeping their own rooms neat and sanitary. Having an orderly room also helped with their mental well-being. Keeping the living spaces healthy also extended to their bodies as students used their extra time working out, practicing yoga, and taking walks. These physical activities were good for their overall physical and mental health. Although the ongoing global pandemic was a psychologically challenging and difficult time for most people, the students showed their resolve, determination, and persistence by working on their academic goals and personal hygiene. In the face of tremendous adversity, they survived and showed their personal resiliency.

## Theme 2: Coping Strategies and Self-Reliance

The second resiliency theme included coping strategies motivated by individual effort or self-reliance. The students explained that part of managing their depressive states or suicide ideation involved beneficial and nourishing practices. Students found resolve in their own abilities to handle and manage psychological challenges. They spent time alone engaging in physical, creative, and reflective activities to reduce the stresses and tensions in their daily lives. They found that these endeavors were healthy for the body, mind, and spirit because they felt stronger overall and more able to cope with negative feelings and emotions. For example, the students found comfort and happiness with physical pursuits such as playing basketball and practicing yoga, in hobbies such as knitting hats and playing guitar, and with reflective pastimes such as reading books and journaling thoughts.

Learning how to live with depression and suicidal thoughts required regular usage of individual coping strategies and efforts developed over the years. Students engaged in other calming and soothing activities to counter undesirable and depressing emotions. They found a sense of peace and tranquility in taking walks with their dogs, studying at a favorite coffee shop, listening to relaxing music, and watching beautiful sunsets. These activities did not necessitate a lot of time but they did have tremendous healing benefits for the students. These individual interests gave them happiness and pleasure. Moreover, the students found that they were not as sad or upset when they remained intentional about these events. These enjoyable activities made living more bearable and worthwhile.

## Theme 3: Support Systems and Human Attachment

The third resiliency theme centered on protective factors in the form of support groups. The two most important support groups were family members and close friends. In these support groups, students did not feel as lonely because they found a place of belonging. Feeling a strong sense of belonging within a community enhanced their feelings for survival. Within the family unit, students embraced the love and contentment from spending time with their younger and older siblings. They found that sharing information and exchanging stories with their siblings were meaningful experiences because spending time together made them feel closer to their siblings. Although students did not discuss their personal problems with their parents, they did feel a sense of security and reassurance knowing their parents were present in their lives. The students described their parents as emotionally unavailable. However, they also expressed a deep appreciation for their parents for providing them with financial support and a place to live. The support from their parents and siblings contributed to their overall willpower to live a productive life.

Most of the students stated that they found strength and endurance in their close friendships. The students reported close friendships with best friends, current roommates, and fraternity or sorority members. The highlight of these friendships was spending time with each other such as watching movies, going out for coffee, and having meals together. The activity itself was not the most important element of the friendship; rather, it was time spent in each other's company and having significant conversations. It was also beneficial for the students to have social relationships with members of their own age group. In general, meaningful friendships made their lives more pleasant and gratifying. Several students attributed their life to their best friends. They acknowledged they are still alive today because their best friends helped them through their darkest moments or days. They expressed their heartfelt and sincere gratitude for the unconditional love, patience, and grace that were given to them in their time of need.

## *Theme 4: Life Skills and Self-Care*

The fourth resiliency theme consisted of life skills in the form of self-care practices. These personal and private routines focused on bettering and enhancing the students. Individually, they developed a sense of empowerment as they made taking care of themselves a high priority. Self-care routines included basic necessities such of hydrating, eating, and sleeping. They made the effort to drink water throughout the day to keep their bodies functioning in a healthy manner. The students were also intentional about reminding themselves to eat throughout the day even though they did not always have an appetite or were too busy with their studies. The need for eating was elevated to a higher level as students selected foods that reminded them of home or when they prepared their own meals with love and care. Some carried on the tradition of cooking special foods for special occasions. Consuming special and delicious rice and soup dishes that reminded them of family and home was also a way of honoring their taste buds. In addition, eating foods that reminded them of their families and homes was comforting for their souls. In this way, eating a special dish from home kept their bodies and souls full and satisfied.

Other self-care practices embraced taking care of the body. Students discussed keeping specific parts of the body clean, including the extra attention they gave to brushing their teeth, taking showers, and clipping their nails. In particular, the special skin care routine allowed students to treat themselves in a loving and gentle manner while also enjoying the end results. Moreover, these collective self-care practices gave the students something to look forward to at the beginning or end of each day. Taking care of themselves was a joyful and pleasurable experience that also increased their self-love and self-respect. These were rituals they performed in the quiet and peace of their personal living spaces. These caring gestures to the self were important ways to connect with one's body. The love and respect they had for themselves made the challenges they experienced in life more bearable and tolerable. Self-care was a form of self-compassion to the students.

### Theme 5: The Accumulation of Good Days

The fifth resiliency theme addressed the importance of accumulated good days for college students. Having a good day is an example of a positive life event. Whereas the accumulation of bad days added an overall sense of heaviness to a student's life, the accumulation of good days contributed to an overall sense of lightness. Thus, the combination of good and bad days made their living journey more balanced. Furthermore, after rough days, the students looked forward to the possibilities of better days ahead. In other words, the moments in a pleasurable day inspired hope for more gratifying days in the future. The feelings of hope contributed to the students' sense of purpose each day. The students stated that a productive day was a good day. They were able to accomplish goals and include a few pleasurable social activities such as spending time with friends or working out.

Moreover, this productive day usually followed a good evening's rest and sleep. Thus, students found that maintaining a schedule and working though their daily tasks contributed to good feelings and well-being throughout the day.

A good day for some students was being able to spend time with their friends. Some were able to spend time with a special friend or a specific group of people on specific days. For example, they might be able to spend time with a special friend because they had classes together throughout the day, or student activity groups to which the students belonged might meet for rehearsal or practice. The anticipation of these special days gave students something to look forward to in the near future. A good day might be the day a student's favorite class meets and the student enjoys the classroom lecture and discussion. The experience of one good day helped students anticipate the possibility of future good days. This future orientation of hope and possibility was a source of optimism, promise, and expectation for the college students. These positive feelings made daily living more meaningful and pleasant. Although the days were not always fully good, students enjoyed the pleasurable moments. Thus, an enjoyable moment gave some balance to the rougher moments.

## Theme 6: Reasons for Living

The sixth and final resiliency theme was remembering the reasons for living. The college students expressed their motivations to live even when they experienced disturbing and disquieting thoughts and emotions. In their reflections, they discussed the importance of individual responsibility as a guiding point for their actions and behaviors. Students conveyed the significance of taking control of their own lives and doing their best to live them meaningfully and productively. They discussed using life-affirming statements as daily reminders to inspire them to work through their mental challenges and difficulties. Words were a source of deep inspiration for the students when they were feeling very down on life. In addition to finding strength in powerful words, students recognized that they were able to survive some of their darkest moments because they had determined and loyal friends by their side. These friends encouraged the students to live by reminding them that their lives have value, meaning, and significance. Furthermore, students found purpose in life through their families. They wanted their family members to be proud of their current academic achievements and future professional accomplishments. Thus, students found strong reasons for living in powerful words, supportive friends, and caring families.

The possibilities that reside in the future were the most important reasons for living. The future held the promise of their dreams and aspirations. Students envisioned achieving their academic goals and, through their professional employment, helping people. They spoke passionately about wanting to help people improve their lives, and the students believed they could make a positive difference in their communities. The future orientation was their goal because it was this forthcoming perspective that kept up their hopes and spirits. Therefore, whereas some students explained that they used their individual determination and ability to move forward, others found the courage and strength to move forward by imagining their future roles of helping other people in need. The potential and promise of the future offered a compelling reason for college students to continue to live with hope.

# The Call for Action

Talking with college students was an enlightening and revelatory experience for me. There is a paradox of mental health vulnerability and resiliency among Asian American college students. I learned that they are vulnerable to suicide ideation but also resilient to suicide death. This is a compelling finding that may be useful and important to systems of higher education as they seek to serve all students using the available human and financial resources on campus. Colleges and universities will want to address the needs of their most vulnerable student populations by creating and maintaining an institutional culture of awareness. Universities that are not currently addressing the specific needs of Asian American college students can use the available research data to better serve this campus population. Specifically, the findings from this study may help institutions of higher education become more aware of the mental health challenges of Asian American college students.

Organizational change is generally not easy to accomplish. Institutions continue to function with familiar practices and are sometimes resistent to new ideas. There may also be a lack of knowledge about how to confront problems in the first place. However, it is important to note that organizational change is imaginable and possible. Colleges and universities are not static establishments; they adjust and adapt to work with the changing needs of their student populations. Ultimately, the needs of college students drive institutional change. Indeed, there should be a goal of helping and supporting the vulnerable campus populations who have mental health challenges succeed as college students.

Colleges and universities want students to succeed by earning their undergraduate degrees. These institutions want all their students to graduate and move forward in their lives. However, Asian American college students have specific vulnerabilities and needs. Addressing the paradox of mental health vulnerability and resiliency among Asian American college students means supporting their pathways to suicide resiliency and developing pathways to lessen their suicide vulnerability. In other words, what can systems of higher education do to help students weaken the risk factors of suicide ideation and strengthen the protective factors of suicide death? To be clear, the systems of higher education are not accountable for every facet of a student's life. For example, they do not have control over a student's bad days or good days. They cannot control the weather or make classes easier. However, they are responsible for creating and maintaining a culture of safety and inclusion.

University administrators, faculty, and staff have an institutional responsibility to create a more welcoming environment for all college students and to generate a greater sense of belonging in the college spaces, including classrooms, residence halls, and open campus areas. When parents send their children to college, there is a general understanding that the university will partially become loco parentis, which refers to the responsibility of an organization to take on some of the functions and responsibilities of a parent.[5] This is particularly true when students are younger than age 18 years. Although college is not the place to parent a child, it does need to nurture young adults as they work on their university degrees. Parents hope that there will be reasonable care and accommodations when they drop off their child at a college or university. They also hope that their child will have access to a variety of available campus support and resources to assist them in their educational endeavors. After all, all students rely on campus resources at some point in their educational journey as they work to achieve their academic goals. For students with mental health vulnerabilities, colleges and universities may need to add more available campus resources. The research findings from this study can help systems of higher education support students who have experienced suicide ideation during their time in college.

## Practice Recommendations

Colleges and universities have the opportunity to make a positive difference in a student's life. There is mounting evidence that mental health struggles and experiences with suicide ideation continue to rise among the college student population. This is a social problem that is not going away soon. The institutional response of silence is not a productive or progressive option because college students are suffering and dying. Systems of higher education are strongly encouraged to take a proactive stance and begin the difficult and important conversation regarding college mental health challenges. One way to begin the conversation with students about suicide ideation and campus resources is to use the academic year to raise awareness about college mental health struggles. In a traditional academic calendar, the fall semester usually begins in August, and the spring semester usually ends in May. September is Suicide Prevention Awareness Month; accordingly, universities may consider providing mental health information and resources to the campus community during this month while students are still enthusiastic about the new term. In addition, this may be a productive time to raise awareness about suicide ideation, suicidal tendencies, and suicide deaths on college campuses. Although this early exchange of information may be raw and difficult, it may also be constructive and beneficial in the long term. Reaching out to students early in the semester sends a message that the university cares about students and wants to take proactive and preventive measures to ensure students' safety and survival. This is a reassuring gesture for students as they see the university taking significant steps to address a serious problem. Receiving information is also helpful to individuals who do not suffer from mental health difficulties because it allows them to be potential advocates for others on campus. Mostly, mental health conversations are useful to remind individuals that they are not alone in their pain and suffering. The message from the university is that *we see you and we will help you in your time of need*. Having initial and timely knowledge regarding psychological well-being has the potential to save lives. Thus, this period of awareness is an opportunity to provide more relevant and needed information to college students.

Providing mental health information to college students early in the semester may also reduce the stigma and silence surrounding experiences with psychological distress. It may offer relief to students who struggle with depression or suicide ideation to know that they are accepted and supported on campus; this will enhance and contribute to feeling a sense of belonging on campus. Reducing a social stigma may also diminish the feelings associated with shame. There should not be feelings of shame associated with being an authentic human being. Moreover, giving voice to an important college crisis that impacts many students requires acts of courage from the campus community to do what is appropriate and necessary for this population. Higher education leaders should not be silent about available psychological and counseling resources. Conversations about mental health struggles and available campus resources may continue throughout the academic year.

May is Mental Health Awareness Month; hence, this might be a good time to continue community outreach regarding mental health issues as students leave campus at the end of the term. It may be useful to provide students with reminders to protect their overall well-being as they separate from the college and university environment. In addition, students should be able to continue to access mental health resources online through the campus website during their summer break. Perhaps universities can provide an accessible summer well-being bundle that students can use while they are off campus. Although it is more difficult to track and monitor undergraduates as they leave campus, it is possible to reach the student population using online tools. Using the academic year to communicate with the student population about the importance of protecting their overall psychological health is a valuable and productive goal.

Although all student populations will benefit from mental health information and services, Asian American college students are particularly vulnerable and have much to gain with the university's messaging and support:

> Because Asian/Pacific Islander and multiracial students are likely to experience concerning psychiatric symptoms and behaviors in the absence of a diagnosis, universities should consider implementing early, proactive, and culturally informed education and prevention programs designed to increase mental health awareness and

engagement, especially among students from these minority backgrounds.[6]

In addition to raising mental health awareness throughout the academic year, there are five pathways to reducing risk factors for suicide ideation and cultivating protective factors against suicide deaths specific to the Asian American student population.

### Practice Recommendation 1: Create a More Inclusive Classroom

Faculty members should be trained and encouraged to create a more inclusive classroom space. Each person benefits when diversity and inclusion are promoted in the classroom. In fact, classes are more engaging and productive when there is a collective sense of belonging and acceptance among students and faculty. This is an important goal because students will spend many hours learning from faculty in the classroom environment. Indeed, students are more likely to have regular contact with the faculty than administrators or staff; thus, faculty members are direct representatives of the campus culture. Often, students believe that the institutional tone of diversity and inclusion is set by the faculty in their classrooms. If they experience perceived racism in the classroom, they will believe that the institution as a whole is also racist. Students have shared with me that professors have been "blatantly racist" in the classroom and that they experienced "backlash standing up to it." It is unclear if some faculty members are intentionally or unintentionally using racist language in the classroom. However, students are often reluctant to confront professors in the moment because they fear the repercussions of social embarrassment and public humiliation. Some students are anxious about how their professors will respond to these delicate situations in the classrooms. This sense of uncertainty generates a high level of discomfort and uneasiness. In some situations, students are afraid to speak up because of the fear of retaliation in the form of lower grades. Furthermore, students are often not aware of any future course of action they may take with the faculty member, academic department, or administrative offices. This renders a sense of powerlessness among Asian American college students. Nevertheless, the students have clearly articulated that faculty should consider creating a more inclusive classroom by understanding their own teaching styles and word choices.

Pedagogy is the art of teaching. There is a strategy to teaching that promotes classroom community engagement. bell hooks, a philosopher and teacher, wrote about the pedagogical importance of creating and maintaining a classroom culture of openness and inclusion in which students could feel a strong sense of belonging. The benefit of feeling a sense of belonging in a classroom context is that a student will feel safe and protected during the learning process. If students believe that they are valued members of the community, they will also engage more fully in that learning community. It is from this safe and protected environment that students can best develop, learn, and feel empowered. This optimal learning space requires the efforts of the entire classroom community who respect and listen to each other: "It has been my experience that one way to build community in the classroom is to recognize the value of each individual voice."[7] Each person in the classroom is encouraged to participate in the scholarly exchange of ideas and experience. There is room for diverse thoughts and there is space for each person, including teachers and students. This position holds that teachers should cultivate student engagement with practices that promote mutual respect and dignity for all classroom members. This includes encouraging—not discouraging—students to use their voices in the classroom.

Each person's voice matters in a college classroom. Students do not just learn from their teachers; they also learn from other students. The college experience supports scholarly debates and personal sharing as important tools for developing understanding and knowledge. Therefore, the classroom culture of sharing is pivotal in the classroom. However, the sharing should be mutual and voluntary, and teachers should set the tone for this respectful community engagement: "In my classroom, I do not expect students to take any risk that I would not take, to share in any way that I would not share."[8] In this manner, the teacher should set the boundaries for acceptable and unacceptable discussion topics. Furthermore, the teacher should convey what is appropriate and inappropriate language in the classroom. Having some guidance and structure will also allow students to know the rules as they participate in thought-provoking and controversial subject matter. There is usually some risk in participating in classroom discussions; however, difficult and challenging conversations can be productive if the classroom culture allows for free thought in a protective and inclusive environment. In this way, teachers should not be the only individuals with a platform to speak.

Teaching and learning are demanding human endeavors. There are high expectations for teachers and students in the classroom; therefore, hooks encourages this learning community to engage in well-being practices. Self-care is beneficial for the teacher and the student: "Teachers must be actively committed to a practice of self-actualization that promotes their own well-being if they are to teach in a manner that empowers students."[9] Teachers and students are human beings, first and foremost, and well-being and empowerment work together in a cycle. When teachers are taking care of their own needs, they will be in a better position to support their students. When students are supported in the classroom, they will develop a sense of empowerment that comes with active classroom engagement. Thus, a professional and caring relationship between faculty and students is desirable and possible. In addition, faculty members as college representatives are in a position to demonstrate that their classroom embraces diversity and supports inclusion. This will go a long way in promoting the mission and vision statements of higher education institutions as places where every student has a place on campus. This is an ambitious goal that will take time to achieve because institutional change is a slow process: "To commit ourselves in the work of transforming the academy so that it will be a place where cultural diversity informs every aspect of our learning, we must embrace struggle and sacrifice."[10]

*Practice Recommendation 2: Participate in Affinity Groups*

The creation of and participation in affinity groups on campus should be encouraged. Student organizations are usually created and run by other students with the support of the campus community. In my interviews, students stated that they felt a strong sense of belonging when they were in the company of other Asian American peoples. There was a feeling of familiarity and comfort when they were in the presence of others who shared their racial and ethnic identity. In the larger campus spaces, they sometimes experienced feelings of difference and isolation; however, when they were around Asian professors, staff, and students, they felt more relaxed and calm. The students felt connected in communities in which there was visible Asian American representation. They credited cultural organizations with a strong Asian American presence as providing a home away from home. Specifically, students expressed the strong sense of belonging that came from a connection with affinity groups. One student stated,

> From a university standpoint as a whole, I felt like I didn't belong at this school but found spaces within the university where I definitely felt a sense of belonging. It was within more Asian American–centric spaces and cultural organization programs where there were Asian American staff or professors.

To meet other Asian American college students with similar backgrounds and interests, students can be encouraged by the student life office to join an existing cultural organization or create a new one. Current student organizations can set up information booths during student orientation week and the early days of the semester. Furthermore, the university website may encourage students to view the student life webpage to learn more about participating in a range of student organizations and activities. If students do not see an existing group they want to join, there should be information on how to create a new student organization on campus. Information on how to form a student group can be shared on the school's website. At the same time, student life leaders may visit residence halls to spread information on the procedures of joining and forming a student organization. Asian Americans are a diverse group representing approximately 50 distinct ethnic groups and speaking more than 30 languages. Thus, Asian Americans are not a monolithic group with the exact same interests, needs, and history. Having an array of affinity groups would honor the diversity of Asian American cultures. As more affinity groups for Asian American college students grow throughout campuses in the United States, there is the possibility of unifying some of these student organizations.

Student organizations on campus can grow into regional conferences with the ability to serve even more students in neighboring cities and states. In 1989, Asian American student leaders from several Midwestern colleges and universities founded the Midwest Asian American Students Union (MAASU) in response to a need for unity among Asian American students in the Midwest. To provide some context of the 1980s, many Asian Americans were trying to make sense of the racially motivated murder of Vincent Chin in Detroit, Michigan, whose killers were never held accountable for the murder after extended legal battles that stretched into the late 1980s. The Chin case highlighted the need to address Asian American civil rights in the United States. As communities throughout the country began organizing around the case to draw attention to continuing racism, college students were inspired to raise concerns about their own experiences with hostile campus climates. As a result, MAASU's founding student leaders came together across the region to create a space for students to examine what it meant to be Asian American living in the United States.[11]

Currently, Asian Americans are living in a similar moment when they are being blamed for the global pandemic. In my conversations with college students, they expressed anger and fear about experiencing racism connected to COVID-19. The deliberate and brazen attacks during Zoom meetings left a chilling effect on the participants. Although some students were not in attendance at these virtual gatherings, they learned about these acts of hate through friends or social media outlets. In their own way, they had to process the anti-Asian sentiments directed at their people. One student stated,

> There was a Zoom call that got bombed by a racist person and I remember that it hit me so hard because—I don't know how to explain it—it's just a feeling that is not easy to describe. I was so furious. That was such an eye opener.

These feelings are reminiscent of when Asian American college students raised issues about racism and a hostile campus environment after the death of Vincent Chin. In the present day, Asian Americans are still grappling with campus racism as they look to each other for strength and solidarity. A student noted,

> I heard it through social sites on social media. I saw it on the news as well. I just heard so many students already saying we stand in solidarity with this cultural group and we are against these racist xenophobic remarks. I'm glad that the community stood up for us.

There is a sense of empowerment in social groups. As the United States confronts another period of hatred and violence against Asian Americans, it is important and necessary to gather together to support Asian communities. A collective group may be a source of strength during these dangerous periods. As Asian Americans are experiencing violence and brutality once again, organizing efforts surge to address the hatred and racism in the country. College students have organized in the past to gain support and solidarity. History repeats itself as Asian Americans organize once again in response to the global pandemic. In the past, forming an Asian American student union gave members a sense of university belonging, including countering racial isolation, establishing

STORIES OF SURVIVAL

a supportive community network, and fostering a sense of solidarity and advocacy through pan-ethnicity.[12] All of these are
needed again as Asian American college students live through the
global pandemic.

*Practice Recommendation 3: Support Family Bonding*

The third recommendation is to support family bonding with institutional resources. Students explained to me that they counted
their immediate family members—parents, brothers, and sisters—
as part of their support system. Although most enjoyed a warm
relationship with their siblings, particularly younger siblings, they
also noted the complicated relationship they had with their parents.
On the one hand, they appreciated their parents' financial support.
On the other hand, they did not feel their parents' emotional support as they experienced college pressures, burdens, and stresses.
Students understood that their parents were greatly concerned
about their academic achievements and successes. However, they
found that their parents were not emotionally available to them.
One student said, "I know that they're there for me no matter what
even though their ways of presenting it may be different or something that I don't prefer, I still know they got my back." Colleges
and universities have the opportunity to support their student
populations by assisting students and parents in enhancing their
communication styles for greater intergenerational connection.
The beginning of the academic year is a productive time to bring
students and their parents together on the college campus. Many
colleges offer parents' weekend programs to bring parents to
campus to learn more about their child's experience. If possible,

colleges may consider offering several parents' weekends over the course of the academic year to include parent–student workshops that focus on different communication styles to enhance family bonding.

Family closeness may take several forms, and there is not just one way for parents and children to connect with each other. Colleges and universities may consider the various ways that parents and students relate to each other within a specific cultural context. For example, some Asian parents may not demonstrate overt expressions of love; rather, warmth and care are often expressed nonverbally and indirectly, such as tending to a student's needs or making sacrifices for the student.[13] Thus, family bonding is not just about parents supporting their children but also about children learning that there are different expressions of parental love and care. Understanding various family dynamics may help colleges develop productive parents' weekends to support the family unit and encourage family cohesiveness. In addition, colleges and universities may consider taking advantage of the first college year to support students and their families. One study focused on the parental role in first-year students' emotional well-being. The research suggested that colleges can use orientation, parent newsletters, counseling, and parent programming to educate students and their parents about the importance of social integration to students' sense of emotional well-being and to help parents and students consider what role parents can play in encouraging their children to make friends and establish a sense of social independence away from home. At the same time, in all interactions with students and parents, institutions should be sensitive to the needs of students from a range of family structures.[14]

## Practice Recommendation 4: Promote Self-Care Practices

The fourth recommendation is to educate all students about the importance of self-care. In general, self-care practices accentuate the positive aspects of health and well-being. Students found expressions of self-love in the activities of self-care. Asian American college students explained that during the first year of the global pandemic, they engaged more in self-care practices. In part, they had more time to engage in activities at home because they were participating in remote learning during the spring and fall semesters. COVID-19 shut down many schools, restaurants, and stores. As a result, students spent time with their families and on themselves. They now had more time and space to engage in self-care routines. They took great care of themselves by continuing to take their medications; learning new ways to cleanse and moisturize their skin; and engaging in physical activities, including skateboarding, playing basketball, and practicing yoga. They found solace and peace in quiet activities such as journaling, reading, and meditating. The students found great comfort in nurturing themselves during this period in the pandemic when people were generally forced to self-quarantine. Although due to the pandemic, people focused more on hygiene, sanitation, and cleanliness, these are also beneficial habits throughout life. Self-care rituals are expressions of self-acceptance, appreciation, and love.

Students explained to me that they were more mindful about the importance of self-care procedures because of their own mental health vulnerabilities. They understood the necessity and value of spending time on themselves because it brought them joy and happiness. They viewed self-care activities as their main responsibility each day while living through the global pandemic. One student stated, "I'm taking care of myself. I should be." Taking care of oneself includes participating in activities that promote overall health and well-being, such as mindfulness, physical exercise, healthy food habits, social support-seeking, and sleep hygiene.[15] As college students with demanding schedules, the process of developing self-care routines is very important. Institutions of higher education have the opportunity to promote the importance of self-care practices among the student population.

There are three pathways to facilitate and promote student self-care practices. First, self-care practices are ideally initiated by students. In this pathway, students must possess the skills of self-awareness, self-help, and self-regulation. Students must learn to be attentive to their physical, psychological, and emotional needs and then generate strategies for meeting those personal needs. However, in some situations, students are not able to identify their self-care needs. They may not know they are able to enhance their overall health and well-being with individual effort. In other situations, students may know they need to engage in healthier practices but may not know about the available options to enhance their overall sense of well-being. For many students, self-care practices need to be enabled, demonstrated, and encouraged by others who are in a position to offer resources and assistance.

Assistance from campus leaders who specialize in student well-being is the second pathway to promote self-care practices. Those who specialize in student well-being may include trained professionals in the areas of health and wellness, mental health and well-being, and psychological and counseling services. These services can provide access to human, electronic, and printed resources relevant to student self-care methods. Furthermore, these advocates for student well-being can offer continuous and ongoing support for students with greater psychological support needs and demands. One such possible initiative is to offer health and well-being coaching delivered by health care professionals with diverse backgrounds. Some students may only need one session, whereas others may need several sessions extended over a period of time. With the assistance of health care professionals, students will be able to access the number of coaching sessions needed for their overall wellness while in college.

The third pathway to facilitate student self-care methods is to include the university community. Self-care processes can be built into core components of the curriculum so that all students are provided with opportunities, guidance, and encouragement to participate in these self-care practices. Requiring students to take a class on self-care and wellness sends a powerful message to the campus community that the university is invested in the full growth and development of all students. The university is making a statement that it supports students' physical and psychological well-being as they work to achieve their educational goals. This broader perspective recognizes the reality that if self-care practices were considered solely as a matter of individual responsibility, it is likely that many students who could benefit from self-care practices would not take advantage of the available resources and training.[16] Therefore, these three pathways support the well-being of the student population with assistance from the university community.

*Practice Recommendation 5: Develop an Asian American Studies Major*

The fifth recommendation is to create and develop an Asian American Studies department that includes a minor, major, and graduate program. In my conversations with students, some expressed their disappointment with the university for not offering Asian American Studies as a major. This lack of presence among academic departments was a reminder to them that their history and culture were not important to the campus community. It sent the message to the students that an Asian American Studies department was not an institutional priority. In addition, it indicated to the students that Asian American experiences were not worth exploring and therefore did not belong on campus. As a result, the students stated that they did not feel a sense of support and belonging on campus. As Asian American college students, they did not feel validated by the university. They did not believe they could celebrate the contributions of Asian Americans to the country. Furthermore, the entire student population did not have the opportunity to learn about the history, culture, and languages of Asian Americans. Moreover, the students shared with me that other racial and ethnic groups had academic departments on campus. One student stated,

> We don't have an Asian American Studies program, whereas we do have a Chicano Studies program, we have an African American program. As a result, I haven't been able to feel as connected to my heritage through the university and through academics as much as other people might.

Building a new major or developing a new academic program takes time. There needs to be personnel to create the curriculum and faculty members who are able to teach these courses. There are standards and procedures to follow in curriculum development, and these steps are generally detail-oriented and time-consuming. However, it is possible and necessity to begin the process of creating a more diverse and inclusive university community by offering more representative academic departments. Examining the creation and development of existing Asian American Studies departments may be useful. Furthermore, it may be useful to understand the history of Asian American identity and struggle as driving forces in developing Asian American Studies departments.

The Asian American pan-ethnic identity grew out of the social justice energy of the mid-20th-century civil rights movements. It was during this period that Asian American activists in the United States fought for the inclusion of their history in the academy. In an attempt to achieve this goal, two critical social movements were born during this period at San Francisco State University (SFSU) in 1968 and University of California, Berkeley (UCB) in 1969. Both campuses went on strike to fight for an ethnic studies program at their universities. Lasting several arduous months, the strikes eventually achieved success with the establishment of the School of Ethnic Studies at SFSU and an Ethnic Studies Department at UCB. Asian American Studies, along with ethnic studies programs nationwide, grew out of these critical movements that were fought hard for by student, faculty, and community activists. Thus, Asian American Studies departments arose out of a strong and collective Asian American identity within the social and historical context of the civil rights movement. Today, Asian American Studies is an institutionalized field in higher education.[17] In 1998, there were 37 Asian American Studies programs; in 2015, there were 53.[18] Scholars have passionately argued that Asian American Studies' central goal and significance have always been to democratize higher education by being part of an effort to change education in all its facets, with an emphasis on making it more equitable, inclusive, and open to alternative perspectives.

Asian American Studies departments are still necessary today. During this time of living through a global pandemic and a rise in anti-Asian hate, Asian American Studies departments have responded to the racialized narrative of the COVID-19 pandemic. Thus, there is a call once again to build Asian American Studies departments in colleges and universities. This time, new Asian American Studies departments may emerge out of a strong and collective Asian American identity within the social and historical context of the global pandemic. Currently, Asian American Studies departments are responding to anti-Asian hate fueled by the ongoing pandemic. Jason Oliver Chang, director of the Asian American studies program at the University of Connecticut, facilitated critical conversations surrounding the virus and its implications in the Asian and Asian American communities. In his essay, he focuses on three main areas of development and concern.

First, the coronavirus was first detected in Wuhan, China, and then rapidly spread to other areas of the world. As it made its way to the United States, it was already being characterized as the Asian virus or the Chinese virus: "The signs that the disease was being characterized in racial terms began to pop up in advance of the virus, because it had clearly arrived in other parts of the world by January."[19] Second, Chang was concerned about news stories during the early months and first year of the global pandemic. He believed that he had a professional and social responsibility to use his training to address and respond to misplaced scapegoating attacks against Asian peoples. In addition, he also needed to publicly respond to the harassment and hate directed against individuals who were perceived to have an Asian background. He remembers this as a dangerous and violent time; however, he was ready to support Asians and Asian Americans as they courageously lived their lives: "We needed to be ready to respond to the mental health and social consequences of anti-Asian racism that could accompany the rise of the virus and potential spread to the United States, which increasingly felt like a distinct possibility."[20]

Finally, Chang believed Asian American Studies departments could offer information and resources as Asians and Asian Americans lived in fear and silence. He was also well aware that his first responsibility was to support the students at his university as they tried to continue their studies during remote learning while facing daily dangers under the umbrella of an uncertain future:

> Faced with rising public anti-Asian violence and harassment, combined with the personal economic strain, loneliness, and difficulties of returning home experienced by so many students, I felt it was more important than ever that the Asian and Asian American Studies Institute answer its mission to serve the UConn Community.[21]

Chang discussed the overall importance and necessity of Asian American Studies programs in responding to the current pandemic:

> The pandemic has animated Asian American studies inside and outside the academy, showing how collective knowledge and wisdom counter xenophobia and racism. Nevertheless, we are confronting the official and popular recuperation of the tired old racial narratives of yellow peril, showing the need to continue walking with Asian American studies. As much as I've been transformed by my education, this experience has shown me that the heart of Asian American studies exists not only in the classroom but also wherever else you take it.[22]

Therefore, an Asian American Studies department has a local and national reach. It can support students when civil rights are under assault, such as during the civil rights movement and in the present time under the global pandemic. It also has a national reach because it offers information and resources to individuals not connected to the university. In this way, one's education and training in Asian American Studies are useful resources when Asian Americans are under attack for merely being Asian Americans. When a university offers an Asian American Studies department, it is supporting its Asian American students and the Asian American community.

## Research Recommendations

My conversations with Asian American college students who have experienced suicide ideation and tendencies took place in the first year of the global pandemic. The students were between ages 18 and 23 years. As I reflect on this process of learning more about suicide vulnerability and resiliency among Asian American college students, I also imagine what more can be done to understand this social phenomenon. What stories am I missing? Who am I missing? In this spirit of reflection and imagination, I offer five research recommendations. First, one way to pivot this research is to focus on international Asian students who study at American universities to determine if they bring a similar or different experience with mental health challenges to college. There is a dearth of research in this particular area; however, there are studies on Chinese students studying at Chinese universities[23] and Korean students studying at Korean universities.[24] Focusing on Asian international students studying at American universities will contribute to more comprehensive knowledge about suicide ideation among the Asian population.

Second, I focused on support systems as a protective factor. Other researchers have found that protective factors might vary as a function of culture.[25] In other words, support systems are not the only protective factors against suicide. There are other concepts of protective factors against suicide ideation and actual suicide, including religion,[26] fear,[27] moral objections,[28] optimism,[29] and positive life events.[30]

Third, future research may focus on transgender Asian American college students. Existing studies on suicide ideation among transgender students focus on lack of seeking mental health support,[31] lack of campus bathroom rights,[32] and lack of campus housing rights.[33] A more specific focus on transgender Asian American college students will contribute to a greater understanding of this diverse student population.

Fourth, I did not focus on college students' gender identities. Future research may focus specifically on suicidal Asian American women who are at risk for interpersonal violence[34] or suicidal Asian American men who experience low self-esteem due to ongoing racial discrimination.[35]

The last research recommendation is to focus specifically on the global pandemic and its impact on Asian American college students' psychological well-being.[36] Connected to this social phenomenon was the rise in anti-Asian hate and violence.[37] These are directly connected to the themes found in this study regarding thwarted belongingness and perceived burdensomeness.

# Conclusion

As long as there are universities, there will be college students. College students come from diverse backgrounds, and some are coming to universities with more mental health challenges than others. As one of the most important stakeholders in higher education, students need more comprehensive mental health resources. There should also be greater awareness about mental health struggles, and there are opportunities in the moment to meet these challenges. Colleges and universities may consider creating more mental health awareness at the beginning and end of the academic year. This could include providing more information about mental health challenges and the services offered on campus. Campuses may also encourage more dialogue about racial tensions and mental health challenges in the classrooms, residence halls, and other campus spaces. Colleges could use resources to support affinity groups and parents' weekends to encourage and develop more support for vulnerable student populations. Furthermore, academic majors can be created to affirm the history of the diverse American population. It is time to examine the organizational culture to understand what students are experiencing so that a more inviting and welcoming environment can be created for all students. Students want to feel a sense of campus, academic, and institutional belonging. It is possible to create a campus environment in which all students, regardless of race or mental health challenges, feel welcomed with a sense of belonging as they work to achieve their educational goals.

# AFTERWORD

My brother died by suicide many years ago. Since his death, I have had time to work through my pain and to process my grief. This is the first time I have publicly addressed my thoughts, feelings, and experiences about this particular piece of my family history with people who do not personally know me. On one level, it is liberating to give voice to my personal suffering because I am sharing an important story about my life. This part of my human journey has helped shaped me into the person that I am today. This is a pivotal piece of who I am as a person. On another level, going back in time to remember the past and to tell it in the present is difficult. There are feeling of distress and sadness. However, I believe it is important to share this part of my life because it may be helpful to see me as not only a teacher and researcher but also a survivor of suicide.

It is difficult to think about my life without also thinking about my brother because he was present for a majority of my years on Earth. When I think back to the year he died, it seems so very long ago. At the same time, it also feels very close to my current life. Remembering my brother, then, is a feeling of both the expansion and compression of time. It is a strange sense to experience diffusion and clarity at the same time. The days after his death were a fog for me. I barely remember going to campus to teach my classes. There are vague memories of conversations regarding the planning of a memorial service. There are hazy recollections of taking care of my family and taking care of myself during this period of deep bereavement. Today, I know that these things did happen because I turned in course grades, attended his memorial service, and my family and I stayed healthy. Although this more recent period remains a blur, going farther back into my early life was more in focus. It was during this time that I thought about what living without my brother would feel like because he was someone I loved very much. Part of the security I felt in this world was the comfort I felt in my brother's presence. My childhood was defined by the things he taught me how to do—throw a football, play basketball, and ride a bicycle. He taught me to enjoy sports and to celebrate the importance of playing. My brother gave me my first baseball mitt, and he helped me shop for a 10-speed bicycle. As kids, my brother took me out for ice cream on my birthday. He helped me move into my college dorm and shop for my first car. As we entered adulthood, we were busy raising our own families in different cities. Still, just knowing that he was a phone call away or that he was still in this world was good enough for me. The world that I lived in always included my brother. Then, one day, he was gone.

The early days without my brother were traumatic and harrowing. I stared at a lot of blank walls in my house, and I cried off and on when I thought about how much he must have suffered. It saddened me to think about how alone he must have felt in this world. Mostly, I just sat with my pain. I cried a lot. I grieved for what felt like a long, long time. My sorrow felt endless. The days became weeks, and the weeks became months. A part of me was robotic and went through the motions of living and responsibilities. It was a joyless time. Each day, it was important to eat food and drink water. Each week, it was important to be present for my family and my work. Each month, it was important to just get through another day. And, when I was able, I wrote in my journal.

Journaling helped me tremendously when I needed to release my confusion or sorrow. It also helped to write about some of our more meaningful experiences together and to celebrate this loving brother–sister relationship. I had very good people who checked in on me and embraced all of me when it was really, really difficult. To be honest, I didn't always feel like talking or sharing my feelings. It was difficult to share feelings when I experienced what I felt was an absence of feelings. I truly felt a deep emptiness that numbed me. It is difficult to explain the void I felt when I was finally able to accept that my brother was no longer alive in this world. I was mourning in a way I have never mourned before. Yet, I always knew that there were loving individuals who would listen to me when I had something to say. My beloved community helped me through this awful period in my life, and they help me still to this day. Loved ones know this part of my life that I don't share with many, and I am deeply grateful for this generous amount of support and love so many years after my brother died. Mostly, the process of time and moving forward with my life helped with my overall healing.

Although my brother's death was not the driving force for me to write this book, I am well aware that he was not far away. I knew my brother was with me while I was doing my work. I hope my brother's death and the many others who die by suicide allow us, as survivors, to grieve and share. If sharing my story and the stories of my participants facilitates this goal, then I am rest assured that this book is meaningful to someone. I am not the first researcher to write a book addressing the suicide of a loved one using my discipline and training as my guide. Thomas Joiner lost his father, Ying-Ying Chang lost her daughter, and Kay Redfield Jamison lost a dear friend. In fact, the book that helped me the most during the first year after my brother's death was *Night Falls Fast: Understanding Suicide* by Kay Redfield Jamison.[1] This book was a saving grace because it helped me understand the history of suicide. In the early days and weeks of mourning and grieving my brother's death, I spent much time in quiet reflection. Having a book guide my thoughts during this painful time in my life aided my healing.

Today, I have made peace with my brother's passing. I miss him, still. I will never truly understand why he died by suicide, but I accept that as a condition of life. There will be mysteries that we cannot solve even though we ask a lot of questions and organize the potential answers. Being able to talk about my brother's death took a long time. I am, by nature and nurture, a reserved and private person. However, I am learning how to better share my stories so that other people can gain some insights into life from my already lived experiences. I think one of the most effective ways to honor those of us who have been touched by suicide ideation or suicide deaths is to offer encouragement to share our stories of struggle and survival. I am deeply inspired by the individuals who have shared their stories of vulnerability and survival with me. Their courage was a tremendous source of inspiration for me to finally share a part of my story. In my classes, I remind myself that I would never ask a student to do something I would not do as a teacher. I am using that same framework and applying it to my work as a researcher with participants. Learning from this group of courageous college students, I hope that we can move forward and continue the conversation on mental health struggles with compassion, understanding, and healing.

# NOTES

## Introduction

1. National Institute of Mental Health. (2022). *Suicide.*
2. Olson, R. (2011). *Suicide and language.* Centre for Suicide Prevention.
3. Centers for Disease Control and Prevention. (2022). *Facts about suicide.* https://www.cdc.gov/suicide/facts/index.html.
4. American Foundation for Suicide Prevention. (2022). *Suicide statistics.* https://afsp.org/suicide-statistics.
5. Schwartz, V. (2016, February). Suicide clusters on college campuses: Risk, prevention, management. *Psychiatric Times, 33*(2).
6. Taub, D. J., & Thompson, J. (2013, Spring). College student suicide. *New Directions for Student Services, 2013*(141), 5–14.
7. Yozwiak, J. A., Lentzch-Parcells, C. M., & Zapolski, T. C. B. (2017). College students and suicide. *International Journal of Child Health and human Development, 10*(4), 311–318.
8. Dueweke, A. R., & Schwartz-Mette, R. A. (2018). Social–cognitive and social–behavioral correlates of suicide risk in college students: Contributions from interpersonal theories of suicide and depression. *Archives of Suicide Research, 22*(2), 224–240.
9. Takaki, R. (1998). *Strangers from a different shore.* Back Bay Books.
10. Pew Research Center. (2021). *Key facts about Asian Americans, a diverse and growing population.* https://www.pewresearch.org/fact-tank/2021/04/29/key-facts-about-asian-americans/#:~:text=Key%20facts%20about%20Asian%20Americans%2C%20a%20diverse%20and%20growing%20population&text=The%20U.S.%20Asian%20population%20is,cultures%2C%20languages%20and%20other%20characteristics.
11. Asian Pacific Institute on Gender-Based Violence. (2019). *U.S. statistics.* https://www.api-gbv.org/resources/census-data-api-identities.
12. Leong, F. T. L., Leach, M. M., Yeh, C., & Chou, E. (2007). Suicide among Asian Americans: What do we know? What do we need to know? *Death Studies, 31*(5), 417–434. https://doi.org/10.1080/07481180701244561.

13. Pew Research Center. (2021). *Key facts about Asian Americans, a diverse and growing population.* https://www.pewresearch.org/fact-tank/2021/ 04/29/key-facts-about-asian-americans/#:~:text=Key%20facts%20ab out%20Asian%20Americans%2C%20a%20diverse%20and%20grow ing%20population&text=The%20U.S.%20Asian%20population%20 is,cultures%2C%20languages%20and%20other%20characteristics.

14. Tran, K. K., Wong, Y. J., Cokley, K. O., Brownson, C., Drum, D., Awad, G., & Wang, M. C. (2015). Suicidal Asian American college students' perceptions of protective factors: A qualitative study. *Death Studies, 39*(8), 500–507. https://doi.org/10.1080/07481187.2014.970299.

15. Sanchez, D., Adams, W. N., Arango, S. C., & Flannigan, A. E. (2018). Racial–ethnic microaggressions, coping strategies, and mental health in Asian American and Latinx American college students: A mediation model. *Journal of Counseling Psychology, 65*(2), 214–225. https://doi. org/10.1037/cou0000249.

16. Wong, J., Brownson, C., Rutkowski, L., Nguyen, C. P., & Becker, M. S. (2014). A mediation model of professional psychological help seeking for suicide ideation among Asian American and White American college students. *Archives of Suicide Research, 18,* 259–273.

17. Choi, J. L., Rogers, J. R., & Werth, J. L., Jr. (2009). Suicide risk assessment with Asian American college students: A culturally informed perspective. *The Counseling Psychologist, 37*(2), 186–218. https://doi.org/ 10.1177/0011000006292256.

18. Centers for Disease Control and Prevention. (2019). *Suicide death rate by race.* https://wisqars.cdc.gov/data/explore-data/explore/selected-years?ex=eyJoYmkiOlsiMCJdLCJpbnRlbnRzIjpbIjAiXSwibWVjaaHM iOlsiMjA4MTAiXSwic3RhdGUiOlsiMDEiLCIwMiIsIjAoIiwiMDUiLC IwNiIsIjA4IiwiMDkiLCIxMCIsIjExIiwiMTIiLCIxMyIsIjE1IiwiMTYiLCI xNyIsIjE4IiwiMTkiLCIyMCIsIjIxIiwiMjIiLCIyMyIsIjI0IiwiMjUiLCIyNi IsIjI3IiwiMjgiLCIyOSIsIjMwIiwiMzEiLCIzMiIsIjMzIiwiMzQiLCIzNSI sIjM2IiwiMzciLCIzOCIsIjM5IiwiNDAiLCI0MSIsIjQyIiwiNDMiLCIoN SIsIjQyIiwiNDciLCIoOCIsIjQ5IiwiNTAiLCI1MSIsIjUzIiwiNTQiLCI1N SIsIjU2IlosInJhY2UiOlsiMSIsIjIiLCIzIiwiNCJdLCJldGGhuaWNoeSI6W ylxIiwiMiIsIjMiXSwic2V4IjpbIjEiLCIyIlosImFnZUdyb3VwcoipbiI6 WyIwMCowNCJdLCJhZ2VHcm91cHNNYXgiOlsiMTk5IlosImN1c3R vbUFnZXNNaW4i4iOlsiMTgiXSwiY3VzdG9tQWdlc01heCI6WyIyNCJ dLCJmcm9tWWVhci6WyIyMDE5IlosInRvWWVhcmI6WyIyMDE5Il osInlwbGwGxBZ2VzIjpbIjYilosIm1ldHJvIjpbIjEiLCIyIlosImFnZWJidH RuIjoiY3VzdG9tIiwiZ3JvdXBieTEiOiJOTo5FIno%3D.

19. Centers for Disease Control and Prevention. (2019). *Suicide death rate by race.* https://wisqars.cdc.gov/data/explore-data/explore/selected-years?ex=eyJoYmkiOlsiMCJdLCJpbnRlbnRzIjpbIjAiXSwibWVjaaHM iOlsiMjA4MTAiXSwic3RhdGUiOlsiMDEiLCIwMiIsIjAoIiwiMDUiLC IwNiIsIjA4IiwiMDkiLCIxMCIsIjExIiwiMTIiLCIxMyIsIjE1IiwiMTYiLCI xNyIsIjE4IiwiMTkiLCIyMCIsIjIxIiwiMjIiLCIyMyIsIjIoIiwiMjUiLCIyNi IsIjI3IiwiMjgiLCIyOSIsIjMwIiwiMzEiLCIzMiIsIjMzIiwiMzQiLCIzNSI sIjM2IiwiMzciLCIzOCIsIjM5IiwiNDAiLCIoMSIsIjQyIiwiNDQiLCIoN SIsIjQ2IiwiNDciLCIoOCIsIjQ5IiwiNTAiLCIhMSIsIjUziiwiNTQiLChiN SIsIjU2Ilos InJhY2UiOlsiMSIsIjIiLCIzIiwiNCJdLCJldGhua WNoeSI6W yIxIiwiMiIsIjMiXSwic2V4IjpbIjEiLCIyIlos ImFnZUdyb3Vwco1pbiI6 WyIwMCowNCJdLCJhZ2VHcm91cHNNNYXgiOlsiMTk5IlosImN1c3R vbUFnZXNNNaW4iOlsiMTgiXSwiY3VzdG9tQWdlc0lheCI6WyIyNCJ dLCJmcm9tWWVhci I6WyIyMDE5IlosInRvWWVhci I6WyIyMDE5Il osInlwbGxwbGxZ2VljpbIjYiXlos Im1ldHJvdXljpbIjEiLCIyIlos ImFnZWJjdH RuLjoiY3VzdG9tIiwiZ3JvdXBieTEiOiJOTo5Fno%3D.

20. Sontag, D. (2002, April 28). Who was responsible for Elizabeth Shin? *The New York Times Magazine.* https://www.nytimes.com/2002/04/28/magazine/who-was-responsible-for-elizabeth-shin.html.

21. McKim, J. B. (2019, September 16). *As student suicides rise, a Harvard case opens new questions about schools' responsibility.* WGBH News, NPR. https://www.wgbh.org/news/education/2019/09/16/as-student-suicides-rise-a-harvard-case-opens-new-questions-about-schools-responsibility.

22. *Woman charged with urging boyfriend to kill himself in "suicide by text" case in Boston.* (2019, October 28). CBS/AP. https://www.cbsnews.com/news/suicide-by-text-inyoung-you-charged-with-urging-boyfriend-alexander-urtula-to-kill-himself.

23. Wang, K. W., Wong, Y. J., & Fu, C. C. (2017). Moderation effects of perfectionism and discrimination on interpersonal factors and suicide ideation. *Journal of Counseling Psychology, 60*(3), 367–378.

24. Reappropriate. (2015). *Asian American student suicide rate at MIT is quadruple the national average.* http://reappropriate.co/2015/05/asian-american-student-suicide-rate-at-mit-is-quadruple-the-national-average.

25. McKim, J. B. (2019, September 16). *As student suicide rises, a Harvard case opens new questions about schools' responsibility.* WGBH News. https://www.wgbh.org/news/education/2019/09/16/as-student-suicides-rise-a-harvard-case-opens-new-questions-about-schools-responsibility.

26. Wong, Y. J., Brownson, C., & Schwing, A. E. (2011). Risk and protective factors associated with Asian American students' suicidal ideation: A multicampus, national study. *Journal of College Student Development, 52*(4), 396–408. https://doi.org/10.1353/csd.2011.0057.

27. Wang, K. W., Wong, Y. J., & Fu, C. C. (2017). Moderation effects of perfectionism and discrimination on interpersonal factors and suicide ideation. *Journal of Counseling Psychology, 60*(3), 367–378.

28. Yozwiak, J. A., Lentzch-Parcells, C. M., & Zapolski, T. C. B. (2017). College students and suicide. *International Journal of Child Health and Human Development, 10*(4), 311–318.

29. Yozwiak, J. A., Lentzch-Parcells, C. M., & Zapolski, T. C. B. (2017). College students and suicide. *International Journal of Child Health and Human Development, 10*(4), 311–318.

30. American Psychiatric Association. (2022). *Diagnostic and statistical manual of mental disorders* (5th ed., text rev.). American Psychiatric Publishing. This is the language found in the DSM; this book does not use the term "committed suicide."

31. Zvolensky, M. J., Jardin, C., Garey, L., Robles, Z., & Sharp, C. (2016). Acculturative stress and experiential avoidance: Relations to depression, suicide, and anxiety symptoms among minority college students. *Cognitive Behaviour Therapy, 45*(6), 501–517. https://doi.org/10.1080/16506073.2016.1205658.

32. Museus, S. D., & Park, J. J. (2015). The continuing significance of racism in the lives of Asian American college students. *Journal of College Student Development, 56*(6), 551–569. https://doi.org/10.1353/csd.2015.0059.

33. Wong, Y. J., Koo, K., Tran, K. K., Chiu, Y.-C., & Mok, Y. (2011). Asian American college students' suicide ideation: A mixed-methods study. *Journal of Counseling Psychology, 58*(2), 197–209. https://doi.org/10.1037/a0023040.

34. Abrams, Z. (2020, July 11). A crunch at college counseling centers. *Monitor on Psychology, 51*(6). https://www.apa.org/monitor/2020/09/crunch-college-counseling.

35. Ruiz, N. G., Edwards, K., & Lopez, M. H. (2021). *One-third of Asian Americans fear threats, physical attacks and most say violence against them is rising.* Pew Research Center. https://www.pewresearch.org/fact-tank/2021/04/21/one-third-of-asian-americans-fear-threats-physical-attacks-and-most-say-violence-against-them-is-rising.

36. Hong, J. C. (2021). *More than 9,000 anti-Asian incidents have been reported since the pandemic began.* The Associated Press. https://www.npr.org/

2021/08/12/1027236499/anti-asian-hate-crimes-assaults-pandemic-incidents-aapi.

37. Stop APPI Hate. (2022). *About Stop APPI Hate.* https://stopaapihate.org.
38. Stop APPI Hate. (2022). *About Stop APPI Hate.* https://stopaapihate.org.
39. Hong, J. C. (2021). *More than 9,000 anti-Asian incidents have been reported since the pandemic began.* The Associated Press. https://www.npr.org/2021/08/12/1027236499/anti-asian-hate-crimes-assaults-pandemic-incidents-aapi.
40. Ruiz, N. G., Edwards, K., & Lopez, M. H. (2021). *One-third of Asian Americans fear threats, physical attacks and most say violence against them is rising.* Pew Research Center. https://www.pewresearch.org/fact-tank/2021/04/21/one-third-of-asian-americans-fear-threats-physical-attacks-and-most-say-violence-against-them-is-rising.
41. Wong, J., Brownson, C., Rutkowski, L., Nguyen, C. P., & Becker, M. S. (2014). A mediation model of professional psychological help seeking for suicide ideation among Asian American and White American college students. *Archives of Suicide Research, 18*(3), 259–273. https://doi.org/10.1080/13811118.2013.824831.
42. Gee, C. B., Khera, G. S., Poblete, A. T., Kim, B., & Buchwach, S. Y. (2020). Barriers to mental health service use in Asian American and European American college students. *Asian American Journal of Psychology, 11*(2), 98–107. https://doi.org/10.1037/aap0000178.
43. Tang, Y., & Masicampo, E. J. (2018). Asian American college students, perceived burdensomeness, and willingness to seek help. *Asian American Journal of Psychology, 9*(4), 344–349. https://doi.org/10.1037/aap0000137.
44. Centers for Disease Control and Prevention. (2019). *Suicide death rate by race.* https://wisqars.cdc.gov/data/explore-data/explore/selected-years?ex=eyJoYmkiOlsiMCJdLCJpbnRlbRzIjpbIjAiXSwibWVjaHM iOlsiMjA4MTAiXSwic3RhdGUiOlsiMDEiLCIwMiIsIjAiIiwiMDUiLC IwNiIsIjA4IiwiMDkiLCIxMCIsIjExIiwiMTIiLCIxMyIsIjE1IiwiMTYiLCI xNyIsIjE4IiwiMTkiLCIyMCIsIjIxIiwiMjIiLCIyMyIsIjI0IiwiMjUiLCIyNi IsIjI3IiwiMjgiLCIyOSIsIjMwIiwiMzEiLCIzMiIsIjMzIiwiMzQiLCIzNSI sIjM2IiwiMzciLCIzOCIsIjM5IiwiNDAiLCIoMSIsIjQyIiwiNDQiLCIoN SIsIjQ2IiwiNDciLCIoOCIsIjQ5IiwiNTAiLCIiMSIsIjUyIiwiNTQiLCIhN SIsIjU2Ilosin jhY2UiOlsiMSIsIjiLCIzIiwiNCJdLCJldGhuaWNoeSI6W yIxIiwiMiIsIjMiXSwic2V4IjpbIjEiLCIyIlosImZnZUdyb3Vwci1bil6 WyIwMCowNCJdLCJhZ2VHcm91cHNNNYXgiOlsiMTk5Ilosim Nic3R vbUFnZXNNaW4iOlsiMTgiXSwiY3VzdG9tQWdlc0iheCI6WyIyNCJ

dLCJmcm9tWWVhciI6WyIyMDE5IlosInRvWWVhciI6WyIyMDE5Il
osInlwbGxBZ2VzIjpbIjY1IlosImildHJvIjpbIjEiLCIyIlosImFnZWJidH
RuIjoiY3VzdG9tIiwiZ3JvdXBieTEiOiJOT05Fno%3D.

45. Asian Pacific Institute on Gender-Based Violence. (2019). *U.S. statistics.*
    https://www.api-gbv.org/resources/census-data-api-identities.
46. Durkheim, E. (1951). *Suicide: A study in sociology.* Free Press. (Original
    work published 1897.)
47. Joiner, T. (2005). *Why people die by suicide.* Harvard University Press.
48. Carrera, S. G., & Wei, M. (2017). Thwarted belongingness, perceived
    burdensomeness, and depression among Asian Americans: A longi-
    tudinal study of interpersonal shame as a mediator and perfection-
    istic family discrepancy as a moderator. *Journal of Counseling Psychology,*
    64(3), 280–291. https://doi.org/10.1037/cou0000199.
49. Van Orden, K. A., Witte, T. K., Cukrowicz, K. C., Braithwaite, S. R.,
    Selby, E. A., & Joiner, T. E. (2010). The interpersonal theory of suicide.
    *Psychological Review,* 117(2), 575–600. https://doi.org/10.1037/a0018697.
50. Van Orden, K. A., Witte, T. K., Cukrowicz, K. C., Braithwaite, S. R.,
    Selby, E. A., & Joiner, T. E. (2010). The interpersonal theory of suicide.
    *Psychological Review,* 117(2), 575–600. https://doi.org/10.1037/a0018697.
51. Young, I. M. (2011). *Justice and the politics of difference.* Princeton University
    Press; p. 53.
52. Wei, M., Yeh, C. J., Chao, R. C., Carrera, S., & Su, J. C. (2013). Family sup-
    port, self-esteem, and perceived racial discrimination among Asian
    American male college students. *Journal of Counseling Psychology,* 60(3),
    453–461. https://doi.org/10.1037/a0032344.
53. Alamilla, S. G., Kim, B. S. K., Walker, T., & Sisson, F. R. (2015).
    Acculturation, enculturation, perceived racism, and psycholog-
    ical symptoms among Asian American college students. *Journal of
    Multicultural Counseling and Development,* 45(1), 37–65. https://doi.org/
    10.1002/jmcd.12062.
54. Nguyen, T. T., Criss, S., Dwivedi, P., Huang, D., Keralis, J., Hsu, E., Phan,
    L., Nguyen, L. H., Yardi, I., Glymour, M. M., Allen, A. M., Chae, D. H.,
    Gee, G. C., & Nguyen, Q. C. (2020). Exploring U.S. shifts in anti-Asian
    sentiment with the emergence of COVID-19. *International Journal of
    Environmental Research and Public Health,* 17(19), 7032. https://doi.org/
    10.3390/ijerph17197032.
55. Le, D., Arora, M., & Stout, C. (2020). Are you threatening me? Asian-
    American panethnicity in the Trump era. *Social Science Quarterly,* 101(6),
    2183–2192. https://doi.org/10.1111/ssqu.12870.

56. Misra, S., Le, P. D., Goldmann, E., & Yang, L. H. (2020). Psychological impact of anti-Asian stigma due to the COVID-19 pandemic: A call for research, practice, and policy responses. *Psychological Trauma: Theory, Research, Practice, and Policy*, 12(5), 461–464. https://doi.org/10.1037/tra 0000821.

57. Carrera, S. G., & Wei, M. (2017). Thwarted belongingness, perceived burdensomeness, and depression among Asian Americans: A longitudinal study of interpersonal shame as a mediator and perfectionistic family discrepancy as a moderator. *Journal of Counseling Psychology*, 64(3), 280–291. https://doi.org/10.1037/cou0000199; Wong, Y. J., Koo, K., Tran, K. K., Chiu, Y.-C., & Mok, Y. (2011). Asian American college students' suicide ideation: A mixed-methods study. *Journal of Counseling Psychology*, 58(2), 197–209. https://doi.org/10.1037/a0023040.

58. Van Orden, K. A., Witte, T. K., Cukrowicz, K. C., Braithwaite, S. R., Selby, E. A., & Joiner, T. E. (2010). The interpersonal theory of suicide. *Psychological Review*, 117(2), 575–600. https://doi.org/10.1037/a0018697.

59. Van Orden, K. A., Witte, T. K., Cukrowicz, K. C., Braithwaite, S. R., Selby, E. A., & Joiner, T. E. (2010). The interpersonal theory of suicide. *Psychological Review*, 117(2), 575–600. https://doi.org/10.1037/a0018697.

60. Wong, Y. J., Koo, K., Tran, K. K., Chiu, Y.-C., & Mok, Y. (2011). Asian American college students' suicide ideation: A mixed-methods study. *Journal of Counseling Psychology*, 58(2), 197–209. https://doi.org/10.1037/a0023040.

61. Wong, Y. J., Brownson, C., & Schwing, A. E. (2011). Risk and protective factors associated with Asian American students' suicidal ideation: A multicampus, national study. *Journal of College Student Development*, 52(4), 396–408. https://doi.org/10.1353/csd.2011.0057.

62. Thapa, P., Sung, Y., Klingbeil, D. A., Lee, C. S., & Klimes-Dougan, B. (2015). Attitudes and perceptions of suicide and suicide prevention messages for Asian Americans. *Behavioral Sciences*, 5(4), 547–564. https://doi.org/10.3390/bs5040547.

63. Carrera, S. G., & Wei, M. (2017). Thwarted belongingness, perceived burdensomeness, and depression among Asian Americans: A longitudinal study of interpersonal shame as a mediator and perfectionistic family discrepancy as a moderator. *Journal of Counseling Psychology*, 64(3), 280–291. https://doi.org/10.1037/cou0000199; Wong, Y. J., Koo, K., Tran, K. K., Chiu, Y.-C., & Mok, Y. (2011). Asian American college students' suicide ideation: A mixed-methods study. *Journal of Counseling Psychology*, 58(2), 197–209. https://doi.org/10.1037/a0023040.

64. Han, M., & Lee, M. (2011). Risk and protective factors contributing to depressive symptoms in Vietnamese American college students. *Journal of College Student Development, 52*(2), 154–166. https://doi.org/10.1353/csd.2011.0032.
65. Wu, G., Feder, A., Cohen, H., Kim, J., Calderon, S., Charney, D., & Mathé, A. A. (2013). Understanding resilience. *Frontiers in Behavioral Neuroscience, 7.* https://doi.org/10.3389/fnbeh.2013.00010.
66. Collins, K. R. L., Stritzke, W. G. K., Page, A. C., Brown, J. D., & Wylde, T. J. (2018). Mind full of life: Does mindfulness confer resilience to suicide by increasing zest for life? *Journal of Affective Disorders, 226,* 100–107. https://doi.org/10.1016/j.jad.2017.09.043; p. 100.
67. University of Southern California. (2019). Lecture notes from Inquiry I class.
68. Zimmerman, M. A. (2013). Resiliency theory: A strengths-based approach to research and practice for adolescent health. *Health Education & Behavior, 40*(4), 381–383. https://doi.org/10.1177/1090198113493782.
69. Cleverley, K., & Kidd, S. A. (2011). Resilience and suicidality among homeless youth. *Journal of Adolescence, 34*(5), 1049–1054. https://doi.org/10.1016/j.adolescence.2010.11.003.
70. Greene, N., Tomedi, L., Reno, J., & Green, D. (2020). The role of substance use and resiliency factors on suicidal ideation among middle school students. *Journal of School Health, 90*(2), 73–80. https://doi.org/10.1111/josh.12854.
71. Sanchez, D., Adams, W. N., Arango, S. C., & Flannigan, A. E. (2018). Racial–ethnic microaggressions, coping strategies, and mental health in Asian American and Latinx American college students: A mediation model. *Journal of Counseling Psychology, 65*(2), 214–225. https://doi.org/10.1037/cou0000249; p. 216.
72. Wu, G., Feder, A., Cohen, H., Kim, J., Calderon, S., Charney, D., & Mathé, A. A. (2013). Understanding resilience. *Frontiers in Behavioral Neuroscience, 7.* https://doi.org/10.3389/fnbeh.2013.00010.
73. Tran, K. K., Wong, Y. J., Cokley, K. O., Brownson, C., Drum, D., Awad, G., & Wang, M. C. (2015). Suicidal Asian American college students' perceptions of protective factors: A qualitative study. *Death Studies, 39*(8), 500–507. https://doi.org/10.1080/07481187.2014.970299.
74. Thapa, P., Sung, Y., Klingbeil, D. A., Lee, C. S., & Klimes-Dougan, B. (2015). Attitudes and perceptions of suicide and suicide prevention messages for Asian Americans. *Behavioral Sciences, 5*(4), 547–564. https://doi.org/10.3390/bs5040547.

75. Wu, G., Feder, A., Cohen, H., Kim, J., Calderon, S., Charney, D., & Mathé, A. A. (2013). Understanding resilience. *Frontiers in Behavioral Neuroscience, 7.* https://doi.org/10.3389/fnbeh.2013.00010.

76. Kleiman, E. M., Riskind, J. H., & Schaefer, K. E. (2014). Social support and positive events as suicide resiliency factors: Examination of synergistic buffering effects. *Archives of Suicide Research, 18*(2), 144–155. https://doi.og/10.1080/13811118.2013.826155.

77. Kleiman, E. M., Riskind, J. H., & Schaefer, K. E. (2014). Social support and positive events as suicide resiliency factors: Examination of synergistic buffering effects. *Archives of Suicide Research, 18*(2), 144–155. https://doi.og/10.1080/13811118.2013.826155.

78. Nayak, A. (2020). *There was a college mental health crisis before COVID-19. Now it may be worse.* Huffington Post. https://www.huffpost.com/entry/college-mental-health-covid-19_l_5f60bec1c5b65fd7b854f1c8.

79. Schwartz, V. (2017). Suicide among college students: Risk and approaches to prevention and management. *Psychiatric Annals, 47*(8), 406–411.

80. Beauchemin, J. D., Facemire, S. D., Pietrantonio, K. R., Yates, H. T., & Krueger, D. (2020). Solution-focused wellness coaching: A mixed methods, longitudinal study with college students. *Social Work in Mental Health, 19*(1), 41–59. https://doi.org/10.1080/15332985.2020.1861165.

81. Dvořáková, K., Greenberg, M. T., & Roeser, R. W. (2018). On the role of mindfulness and compassion skills in students' coping, well-being, and development across the transition to college: A conceptual analysis. *Stress and Health, 35*(2), 146–156. https://doi.org/10.1002/smi.2850.

82. Seidman, I. (2019). *Interviewing as qualitative research: A guide for researchers in education and the social sciences.* Teachers College Press.

83. Merriam, S. B., & Tisdell, E. J. (2016). *Qualitative research: A guide to design and implementation.* Jossey-Bass.

84. Creswell, J. W. (2014). *Research design: Qualitative, quantitative, and mixed method approaches.* SAGE.

85. Creswell, J. W., & Creswell, J. D. (2018). *Research design: Qualitative, quantitative, and mixed method approaches.* SAGE.

86. Smith, L. T. (2012). *Decolonizing methodologies: Research and Indigenous peoples.* Zed Books.

87. Smith, L. T. (2012). *Decolonizing methodologies: Research and Indigenous peoples.* Zed Books; p. 146.

88. Ravitch, S. M., & Carl, N. M. (2021). *Qualitative research: Bridging the conceptual, theoretical, and methodological.* SAGE.

89. Creswell, J. W., & Poth, C. N. (2018). *Qualitative inquiry and research design: Choosing among five approaches*. SAGE.

90. Tuck, E., & Yang, K. W. (2014). R-words: Refusing research. In D. Paris & M. T. Winn (Eds.), Humanizing research: Decolonizing qualitative inquiry with youth and communities (pp. 223–248). SAGE.

91. Rosenberg, S. (2017). *Respective collection of demographic data*. https://medium.com/@anna.sarai.rosenberg/respectful-collection-of-demographic-data-56de9fcb80e2.

# Chapter 1

1. Jackson, J. (2022). *A handbook for survivors of suicide*. American Association of Suicidology. https://suicidology.org/wp-content/uploads/2019/07/SOS_handbook.pdf; p. 9.

2. American Psychological Association. (2022). *Binge-eating disorder*. https://dictionary.apa.org/binge-eating-disorder.

3. Vuong, O. (2019). *On earth we're briefly gorgeous*. Penguin.

4. Carrera, S. G., & Wei, M. (2017). Thwarted belongingness, perceived burdensomeness, and depression among Asian Americans: A longitudinal study of interpersonal shame as a mediator and perfectionistic family discrepancy as a moderator. *Journal of Counseling Psychology, 64*(3), 280–291. https://doi.org/10.1037/cou0000199.

5. Samura, M. (2016). Remaking selves, repositioning selves, or remaking space: An examination of Asian American college students' processes of "belonging." *Journal of College Student Development, 57*(2), 135–150. https://doi.org/10.1353/csd.2016.0016.

6. Choi, J. L., & Rogers, J. R. (2010). Exploring the validity of the College Student Reasons for Living Inventory among Asian American college students. *Archives of Suicide Research, 14*(3), 222–235. https://doi.org/10.1080/13811118.2010.494135.

7. Gadsby, S. (2022). Imposter syndrome and self-deception. *Australasian Journal of Philosophy, 100*(2), 247–261. https://doi.org/10.1080/00048402.2021.1874445.

8. Hong, J. C. (2021, August 12). *More than 9,000 anti-Asian incidents have been reported since the pandemic began*. The Associated Press. https://www.npr.org/2021/08/12/1027236499/anti-asian-hate-crimes-assaults-pandemic-incidents-aapi.

9. Hong, J. C. (2021, August 12). *More than 9,000 anti-Asian incidents have been reported since the pandemic began.* The Associated Press. https://www.npr.org/2021/08/12/1027236499/anti-asian-hate-crimes-assaults-pandemic-incidents-aapi.

10. Kim, P. Y., Kendall, D. L., & Cheon, H. (2017). Racial microaggressions, cultural mistrust, and mental health outcomes among Asian American college students. *American Journal of Orthopsychiatry, 87*(6), 663–670. https://doi.org/10.1037/ort0000203; p. 663

11. Sanchez, D., Adams, W. N., Arango, S. C., & Flannigan, A. E. (2018). Racial–ethnic microaggressions, coping strategies, and mental health in Asian American and Latinx American college students: A mediation model. *Journal of Counseling Psychology, 65*(2), 214–225. https://doi.org/10.1037/cou0000249.

12. Kendi, I. X. (2019). *How to be an antiracist.* Random House.

13. Gordon, J. S. (2019). *The transformation: Discovering wholeness and healing after trauma.* HarperOne.

14. Tummala-Narra, P., Li, Z., Chang, J., Yang, E. J., Jiang, J., Sagherian, M., Phan, J., & Alfonso, A. (2018). Developmental and contextual correlates of mental health and help-seeking among Asian American college students. *American Journal of Orthopsychiatry, 88*(6), 636–649. https://doi.org/10.1037/ort0000317.

15. Poon, O., Squire, D., Kodama, C., Byrd, A., Chan, J., Manzano, L., Furr, S., & Bishundat, D. (2016). A critical review of the model minority myth in selected literature on Asian Americans and Pacific Islanders in higher education. *Review of Educational Research, 86*(2), 469–502. https://doi.org/10.3102/0034654315612205.

16. Tran, K. K., Wong, Y. J., Cokley, K. O., Brownson, C., Drum, D., Awad, G., & Wang, M. C. (2015). Suicidal Asian American college students' perceptions of protective factors: A qualitative study. *Death Studies, 39*(8), 500–507. https://doi.org/10.1080/07481187.2014.970299.

17. Takaki, R. (1998). *Strangers from a different shore.* Back Bay Books.

18. Tummala-Narra, P., Li, Z., Chang, J., Yang, E. J., Jiang, J., Sagherian, M., Phan, J., & Alfonso, A. (2018). Developmental and contextual correlates of mental health and help-seeking among Asian American college students. *American Journal of Orthopsychiatry, 88*(6), 636–649. https://doi.org/10.1037/ort0000317.

19. Perez, M. A., Santos, A. A., Cisneros, R., & Tongson-Fernandez, M. (2019). Stress, stressors, and academic performance among Asian students in central California. *American Journal of Health Studies, 34*(1), 29.

20. Carrera, S. G., & Wei, M. (2017). Thwarted belongingness, perceived burdensomeness, and depression among Asian Americans: A longitudinal study of interpersonal shame as a mediator and perfectionistic family discrepancy as a moderator. *Journal of Counseling Psychology*, 64(3), 280–291. https://doi.org/10.1037/cou0000199; Wong, Y. J., Koo, K., Tran, K. K., Chiu, Y.-C., & Mok, Y. (2011). Asian American college students' suicide ideation: A mixed-methods study. *Journal of Counseling Psychology*, 58(2), 197–209. https://doi.org/10.1037/a0023040.

21. Choi, J. L., Rogers, J. R., & Werth, J. L., Jr. (2009). Suicide risk assessment with Asian American college students: A culturally informed perspective. *The Counseling Psychologist*, 37(2), 186–218. https://doi.org/10.1177/0011000006292256.

22. Samura, M. (2015). Wrestling with expectations: An examination of how Asian American college students negotiate personal, parental, and societal expectations. *Journal of College Student Development*, 56(6), 602–618. https://doi.org/10.1353/csd.2015.0065.

23. Wong, Y. J., Brownson, C., & Schwing, A. E. (2011). Risk and protective factors associated with Asian American students' suicidal ideation: A multicampus, national study. *Journal of College Student Development*, 52(4), 396–408. https://doi.org/10.1353/csd.2011.0057.

24. Perez, M. A., Santos, A. A., Cisneros, R., & Tongson-Fernandez, M. (2019). Stress, stressors, and academic performance among Asian students in central California. *American Journal of Health Studies*, 34(1), 29.

25. Choi, J. L., Rogers, J. R., & Werth, J. L., Jr. (2009). Suicide risk assessment with Asian American college students: A culturally informed perspective. *The Counseling Psychologist*, 37(2), 186–218. https://doi.org/10.1177/0011000006292256.

# Chapter 2

1. Centers for Disease Control and Prevention. (2017). *Preventing suicide: A technical package of policies, programs, and practice.* http://dx.doi.org/10.15620/cdc.44275.

2. Centers for Disease Control and Prevention. (2017). *Preventing suicide: A technical package of policies, programs, and practice.* http://dx.doi.org/10.15620/cdc.44275.

3. Therapist Aid. (2021). *Protective factors.* https://www.therapistaid.com/worksheets/protective-factors.pdf.

4. Substance Abuse and Mental Health Services Administration. (2021). *Risk and protective factors.* https://www.samhsa.gov/sites/default/files/20190718-samhsa-risk-protective-factors.pdf.

5. Nayak, A. (2020). *There was a college mental health crisis before COVID-19. Now it may be worse.* Huffington Post. https://www.huffpost.com/entry/college-mental-health-covid-19_l_5f60bec1c5b65fd7b854f1c8.

6. Abrams, Z. (2020). A crunch at college counseling centers. *Monitor on Psychology, 51*(6).

7. Abrams, Z. (2020). A crunch at college counseling centers. *Monitor on Psychology, 51*(6).

8. Tran, K. K., Wong, Y. J., Cokley, K. O., Brownson, C., Drum, D., Awad, G., & Wang, M. C. (2015). Suicidal Asian American college students' perceptions of protective factors: A qualitative study. *Death Studies, 39*(8), 500–507. https://doi.org/10.1080/07481187.2014.970299.

9. Tran, K. K., Wong, Y. J., Cokley, K. O., Brownson, C., Drum, D., Awad, G., & Wang, M. C. (2015). Suicidal Asian American college students' perceptions of protective factors: A qualitative study. *Death Studies, 39*(8), 500–507. https://doi.org/10.1080/07481187.2014.970299.

10. Wu, G., Feder, A., Cohen, H., Kim, J., Calderon, S., Charney, D., & Mathé, A. A. (2013). Understanding resilience. *Frontiers in Behavioral Neuroscience, 7.* https://doi.org/10.3389/fnbeh.2013.00010.

11. Wong, Y. J., Brownson, C., & Schwing, A. E. (2011). Risk and protective factors associated with Asian American students' suicidal ideation: A multicampus, national study. *Journal of College Student Development, 52*(4), 396–408. https://doi.org/10.1353/csd.2011.0057.

12. Collins, K. R. L., Stritzke, W. G. K., Page, A. C., Brown, J. D., & Wylde, T. J. (2018). Mind full of life: Does mindfulness confer resilience to suicide by increasing zest for life? *Journal of Affective Disorders, 226,* 100–107. https://doi.org/10.1016/j.jad.2017.09.043.

13. Collins, K. R. L., Stritzke, W. G. K., Page, A. C., Brown, J. D., & Wylde, T. J. (2018). Mind full of life: Does mindfulness confer resilience to suicide by increasing zest for life? *Journal of Affective Disorders, 226,* 100–107. https://doi.org/10.1016/j.jad.2017.09.043.

14. Maslow, A. H. (2013). *A theory of motivation.* Martino.

15. Wu, G., Feder, A., Cohen, H., Kim, J., Calderon, S., Charney, D., & Mathé, A. A. (2013). Understanding resilience. *Frontiers in Behavioral Neuroscience, 7.* https://doi.org/10.3389/fnbeh.2013.00010.

16. Wong, Y. J., Brownson, C., & Schwing, A. E. (2011). Risk and protective factors associated with Asian American students' suicidal ideation: A

multicampus, national study. *Journal of College Student Development, 52*(4), 396–408. https://doi.org/10.1353/csd.2011.0057.

17. Schwartz, V. (2017). Suicide among college students: Risk and approaches to prevention and management. *Psychiatric Annals, 47*(8), 406–411.

18. Moses, J., Bradley, G. L., & O'Callaghan, F. V. (2016). When college students look after themselves: Self-care practices and well-being. *Journal of Student Affairs Research and Practice, 53*(3), 346–359.

19. Beauchemin, J. D., Facemire, S. D., Pietrantonio, K. R., Yates, H. T., & Krueger, D. (2020). Solution-focused wellness coaching: A mixed methods, longitudinal study with college students. *Social Work in Mental Health, 19*(1), 41–59. https://doi.org/10.1080/15332985.2020.1861165.

20. Nayak, A. (2020). *There was a college mental health crisis before COVID-19. Now it may be worse.* Huffington Post. https://www.huffpost.com/entry/college-mental-health-covid-19_l_5f60bec1c5b65fd7b854f1c8.

21. Beauchemin, J. D., Facemire, S. D., Pietrantonio, K. R., Yates, H. T., & Krueger, D. (2020). Solution-focused wellness coaching: A mixed methods, longitudinal study with college students. *Social Work in Mental Health, 19*(1), 41–59. https://doi.org/10.1080/15332985.2020.1861165.

22. Dvořáková, K., Greenberg, M. T., & Roeser, R. W. (2018). On the role of mindfulness and compassion skills in students' coping, well–being, and development across the transition to college: A conceptual analysis. *Stress and Health, 35*(2), 146–156. https://doi.org/10.1002/smi.2850.

23. Nayak, A. (2020). *There was a college mental health crisis before COVID-19. Now it may be worse.* Huffington Post. https://www.huffpost.com/entry/college-mental-health-covid-19_l_5f60bec1c5b65fd7b854f1c8.

24. Kleiman, E. M., Riskind, J. H., & Schaefer, K. E. (2014). Social support and positive events as suicide resiliency factors: Examination of synergistic buffering effects. *Archives of Suicide Research, 18*(2), 144–155. https://doi.org/10.1080/13811118.2013.826155.

25. Thapa, P., Sung, Y., Klingbeil, D. A., Lee, C. S., & Klimes-Dougan, B. (2015). Attitudes and perceptions of suicide and suicide prevention messages for Asian Americans. *Behavioral Sciences, 5*(4), 547–564. https://doi.org/10.3390/bs5040547.

26. Kleiman, E. M., & Beaver, J. K. (2013). A meaningful life is worth living: Meaning in life as a suicide resiliency factor. *Psychiatry Research, 210*(3), 934–939. https://doi.org/10.1016/j.psychres.2013.08.002.

27. Kleiman, E. M., & Beaver, J. K. (2013). A meaningful life is worth living: Meaning in life as a suicide resiliency factor. *Psychiatry Research*, 210(3), 934–939. https://doi.org/10.1016/j.psychres.2013.08.002.
28. Tran, K. K., Wong, Y. J., Cokley, K. O., Brownson, C., Drum, D., Awad, G., & Wang, M. C. (2015). Suicidal Asian American college students' perceptions of protective factors: A qualitative study. *Death Studies*, 39(8), 500–507. https://doi.org/10.1080/07481187.2014.970299.
29. Cited in Tran, K. K., Wong, Y. J., Cokley, K. O., Brownson, C., Drum, D., Awad, G., & Wang, M. C. (2015). Suicidal Asian American college students' perceptions of protective factors: A qualitative study. *Death Studies*, 39(8), 500–507. https://doi.org/10.1080/07481187.2014.970299.
30. Choi, J. L., & Rogers, J. R. (2010). Exploring the validity of the College Student Reasons for Living Inventory among Asian American college students. *Archives of Suicide Research*, 14(3), 222–235. https://doi.org/10.1080/13811118.2010.494135.

# Chapter 3

1. Johnson, M., Flynn, E., & Monroe, M. (2016). A residence plan for success for at-risk college students: Reviving "in loco parentis." *College Student Journal*, 50(2), 268–274.
2. Johnson, M., Flynn, E., & Monroe, M. (2016). A residence plan for success for at-risk college students: Reviving "in loco parentis." *College Student Journal*, 50(2), 268–274.
3. Alamilla, S. G., Kim, B. S. K., Walker, T., & Sisson, F. R. (2015). Acculturation, enculturation, perceived racism, and psychological symptoms among Asian American college students. *Journal of Multicultural Counseling and Development*, 45(1), 37–65. https://doi.org/10.1002/jmcd.12062; Augsberger, A., Rivera, A. M., Hahm, C. T., Lee, Y. A., Choi, Y., & Hahm, H. C. (2018). Culturally related risk factors of suicidal ideation, intent, and behavior among Asian American women. *Asian American Journal of Psychology*, 9(4), 252–261. https://doi.org/10.1037/aap0000146; Carrera, S. G., & Wei, M. (2017). Thwarted belongingness, perceived burdensomeness, and depression among Asian Americans: A longitudinal study of interpersonal shame as a mediator and perfectionistic family discrepancy as a moderator. *Journal of Counseling Psychology*, 64(3), 280–291. https://doi.org/10.1037/cou0000199; Leong, F. T. L., Chu, J., & Joshi, S. V. (2018). Guest editors'

introduction to special issue on advancing our understanding of suicide among Asian Americans. *Asian American Journal of Psychology,* 9(4), 247–251. https://doi.org/10.1037/aap0000148; Sa, J., Choe, C. S., Cho, C. B., Chaput, J., Lee, J., & Hwang, S. (2020). Sex and racial/ethnic differences in suicidal consideration and suicide attempts among US college students, 2011–2015. *American Journal of Health Behavior,* 44(2), 214–231. https://doi.org/10.5993/AJHB.44.2.9; Tang, Y., & Masicampo, E. J. (2018). Asian American college students, perceived burdensomeness, and willingness to seek help. *Asian American Journal of Psychology,* 9(4), 344–349. https://doi.org/10.1037/aap0000137.

4. Mackenzie, S., Wiegel, J. R., Mundt, M., Brown, D., Saewyc, E., Heiligenstein, E., Harahan, B., & Fleming, M. (2011). Depression and suicide ideation among students accessing campus health care. *American Journal of Orthopsychiatry,* 81(1), 101–107. https://doi.org/10.1111/j.1939-0025.2010.01077.x.

5. Sax, L. J., & Weintraub, D. S. (2014). Exploring the parental role in first-year students' emotional well-being: Considerations by gender. *Journal of Student Affairs Research and Practice,* 51(2), 113–127. https://doi.org/10.1515/jsarp-2014-0013.

6. Chen, J. A., Stevens, C., Wong, S. H. M., & Liu, C. H. (2019). Psychiatric symptoms and diagnoses among U.S. college students: A comparison by race and ethnicity. *Psychiatric Services,* 70(6), 442–449. https://doi.org/10.1176/appi.ps.201800388; p. 447.

7. hooks, b. (1994). *Teaching to transgress: Education as the practice of freedom.* Routledge; p. 40.

8. hooks, b. (1994). *Teaching to transgress: Education as the practice of freedom.* Routledge; p. 21.

9. hooks, b. (1994). *Teaching to transgress: Education as the practice of freedom.* Routledge; p. 15.

10. hooks, b. (1994). *Teaching to transgress: Education as the practice of freedom.* Routledge; p. 33.

11. Kodama, C. M., Poon, O. A., Manzano, L. J., & Sihite, E. U. (2017). Geographic constructions of race: The Midwest Asian American students union. *Journal of College Student Development,* 58(6), 872–890. https://doi.org/10.1353/csd.2017.0069.

12. Kodama, C. M., Poon, O. A., Manzano, L. J., & Sihite, E. U. (2017). Geographic constructions of race: The Midwest Asian American students union. *Journal of College Student Development,* 58(6), 872–890. https://doi.org/10.1353/csd.2017.0069.

13. Choi, Y., Park, M., Lee, J. P., & Lee, M. (2020). Explaining the Asian American youth paradox: Universal factors versus Asian American family process among Filipino and Korean American youth. *Family Processes, 59*(4), 1818–1836.

14. Sax, L. J., & Weintraub, D. S. (2014). Exploring the parental role in first-year students' emotional well-being: Considerations by gender. *Journal of Student Affairs Research and Practice, 51*(2), 113–127. https://doi.org/10.1515/jsarp-2014-0013.

15. Moses, J., Bradley, G. L., & O'Callaghan, F. V. (2016). When college students look after themselves: Self-care practices and well-being. *Journal of Student Affairs Research and Practice, 53*(3), 346–359.

16. Moses, J., Bradley, G. L., & O'Callaghan, F. V. (2016). When college students look after themselves: Self-care practices and well-being. *Journal of Student Affairs Research and Practice, 53*(3), 346–359.

17. Trieu, M. M. (2018). "It was about claiming space": Exposure to Asian American studies, ethnic organization participation, and the negotiation of self among southeast Asian Americans. *Race, Ethnicity and Education, 21*(4), 518–539. https://doi.org/10.1080/13613324.2016.1272564.

18. Trieu, M. M. (2018). "It was about claiming space": Exposure to Asian American studies, ethnic organization participation, and the negotiation of self among southeast Asian Americans. *Race, Ethnicity and Education, 21*(4), 518–539. https://doi.org/10.1080/13613324.2016.1272564.

19. Chang, J. O. (2020). Walking with Asian American studies. *Journal of Asian American Studies, 23*(3), 329–333. https://doi.org/10.1353/jaas.2020.0026; p. 329.

20. Chang, J. O. (2020). Walking with Asian American studies. *Journal of Asian American Studies, 23*(3), 329–333. https://doi.org/10.1353/jaas.2020.0026; p. 330.

21. Chang, J. O. (2020). Walking with Asian American studies. *Journal of Asian American Studies, 23*(3), 329–333. https://doi.org/10.1353/jaas.2020.0026; p. 331.

22. Chang, J. O. (2020). Walking with Asian American studies. *Journal of Asian American Studies, 23*(3), 329–333. https://doi.org/10.1353/jaas.2020.0026; p. 333.

23. Wang, L., He, C. Z., Yu, Y. M., Qiu, X. H., Yang, X. X., Qiao, Z. X., Sui, H., Zhu, X. Z., & Yang, Y. J. (2014). Associations between impulsivity, aggression, and suicide in Chinese college students. *BMC Public Health, 14*(1), Article 551. https://doi.org/10.1186/1471-2458-14-551.

24. Lee, Y., & Oh, K. J. (2012). Validation of reasons for living and their relationship with suicidal ideation in Korean college students. *Death Studies, 36*(8), 712–722. https://doi.org/10.1080/07481187.2011.584011.

25. Choi, J. L., & Rogers, J. R. (2010). Exploring the validity of the College Student Reasons for Living Inventory among Asian American college students. *Archives of Suicide Research, 14*(3), 222–235. https://doi.org/10.1080/13811118.2010.494135.

26. Wong, Y. J., Brownson, C., & Schwing, A. E. (2011). Risk and protective factors associated with Asian American students' suicidal ideation: A multicampus, national study. *Journal of College Student Development, 52*(4), 396–408. https://doi.org/10.1353/csd.2011.0057; Kim, P. Y., Kendall, D. L., & Webb, M. (2015). Religious coping moderates the relation between racism and psychological well-being among Christian Asian American college students. *Journal of Counseling Psychology, 62*(1), 87–94. https://doi.org/10.1037/cou0000055.

27. Tran, K. K., Wong, Y. J., Cokley, K. O., Brownson, C., Drum, D., Awad, G., & Wang, M. C. (2015). Suicidal Asian American college students' perceptions of protective factors: A qualitative study. *Death Studies, 39*(8), 500–507. https://doi.org/10.1080/07481187.2014.970299.

28. Choi, J. L., & Rogers, J. R. (2010). Exploring the validity of the College Student Reasons for Living Inventory among Asian American college students. *Archives of Suicide Research, 14*(3), 222–235. https://doi.org/10.1080/13811118.2010.494135.

29. Yu, E. A., & Chang, E. C. (2016). Optimism/pessimism and future orientation as predictors of suicidal ideation: Are there ethnic differences? *Cultural Diversity & Ethnic Minority Psychology, 22*(4), 572–579. https://doi.org/10.1037/cdp0000107.

30. Kleiman, E. M., Riskind, J. H., & Schaefer, K. E. (2014). Social support and positive events as suicide resiliency factors: Examination of synergistic buffering effects. *Archives of Suicide Research, 18*(2), 144–155. https://doi.og/10.1080/13811118.2013.826155.

31. Oswalt, S., & Lederer, A. (2017). Beyond depression and suicide: The mental health of transgender college students. *Social Sciences, 6*(1), 1–10. https://doi.org/10.3390/socsci6010020.

32. Sutton, H. (2016). Transgender college students more at risk for suicide when denied bathroom, housing rights. *Campus Security Report, 13*(2), 9. https://doi.org/10.1002/casr.30167.

33. Seelman, K. L. (2016). Transgender adults' access to college bathrooms and housing and the relationship to suicidality. *Journal of Homosexuality*, *63*(10), 1378–1399. https://doi.org/10.1080/00918369.2016.1157998.

34. Augsberger, A., Yeung, A., Dougher, M., & Hahm, H. C. (2015). Factors influencing the underutilization of mental health services among Asian American women with a history of depression and suicide. *BMC Health Services Research*, *15*(1), Article 542. https://doi.org/10.1186/s12913-015-1191-7.

35. Wei, M., Yeh, C. J., Chao, R. C., Carrera, S., & Su, J. C. (2013). Family support, self-esteem, and perceived racial discrimination among Asian American male college students. *Journal of Counseling Psychology*, *60*(3), 453–461. https://doi.org/10.1037/a0032344.

36. Misra, S., Le, P. D., Goldmann, E., & Yang, L. H. (2020). Psychological impact of anti-Asian stigma due to the COVID-19 pandemic: A call for research, practice, and policy responses. *Psychological Trauma*, *12*(5), 461–464. https://doi.org/10.1037/tra0000821.

37. Le, D., Arora, M., & Stout, C. (2020). Are you threatening me? Asian-American panethnicity in the Trump era. *Social Science Quarterly*, *101*(6), 2183–2192. https://doi.org/10.1111/ssqu.12870; Nguyen, T. T., Criss, S., Dwivedi, P., Huang, D., Keralis, J., Hsu, E., Phan, L., Nguyen, L. H., Yardi, I., Glymour, M. M., Allen, A. M., Chae, D. H., Gee, G. C., & Nguyen, Q. C. (2020). Exploring U.S. shifts in anti-Asian sentiment with the emergence of COVID-19. *International Journal of Environmental Research and Public Health*, *17*(19), 7032. https://doi.org/10.3390/ijerph17197032.

# Afterword

1. Redfield Jamison, K. (1999). Night falls fast. Knopf.

# INDEX

*For the benefit of digital users, indexed terms that span two pages (e.g., 52–53) may, on occasion, appear on only one of those pages.*

Tables, figures, and boxes are indicated by *t, f,* and *b* following the page number

abuse
  at home, 117, 150
  intergenerational transmission
    of, 49–50
  racist, 67
academic achievement
  false assumptions about Asian
    Americans and, 66
  parental expectations for, 74–75,
    77, 79–80
academic calendar, and raising
    awareness about mental
    health, 172–75
academic challenges. *See also*
    academic pressures
  global pandemic and, 42
academic competition, 59–60, 154
academic pressures, 14, 22, 41,
    57–60, 84–85, 158
  in middle and high school, 34–
    35, 149
acceptance, as coping mechanism, 111
acculturation, 12–13. *See also* cultural
    challenges
addictive disorders, 37

affinity groups. *See also* student
    organizations
  participation in (practice
    recommendation), 178–82
age, and suicide death rate, 18
alienation, pressure for academic
    achievement and, 80
ambiguous loss, 94
anti-Asian incidents/hate/violence,
    62, 147, 181–82, 189–90
  pandemic and, 15–16, 21 (*see also*
    COVID-19)
  research on, recommendations
    for, 192
anxiety, 12, 38–39, 160–61
  in pandemic, 162–63
  pandemic and, 93–94
Asian American college students,
    2–3. *See also* research
    participants
  gender identity, and suicide risk,
  research on, recommendations
    for, 192
  mental health awareness
    programs for, 174–75

Asian American college students
(*cont.*)
and mental health support,
17, 39–40
as percentage of college
population, 8–9, 65
population growth, 7
social experiences of, and mental
health challenges, 12–16
stereotyping of, 66, 69–70, 154–55
suicidal ideation in, 7–8, 12, 18–23
suicide death rate in, 7–9
suicide resiliency in, 146–47
suicides, media coverage of, 8–9
suicide vulnerability, 145–47
transgender, research on,
recommendations for, 192
Asian American identity, 188–89
Asian Americans, 2
as COVID-19 scapegoats, 15–16,
62–63, 154–55, 157–58, 180–81
cultural norms, and perceived
burdensomeness, 81
as diverse and distinct group, 7
ethnicity and national origin of,
6f, 6–7
hate crimes against, 21
population growth, 7
suicide death rates in, 19t
U.S. Census Bureau
classification of, 18
Asian American Studies program
development of (practice
recommendation), 186–91
lack of, 69–70, 156–57
pandemic and, 189–90
Asian international students,
at American universities,
research on, 191–92

attachment. *See* human attachment
awareness
institutional culture of, 170–72
mental health, raising,
throughout academic
year, 172–91

bad day(s), 31–32, 92
accumulation of, 148, 151–52
and good days, balance of, 139–
40, 167–68
and mental health struggles, 40–
46, 148
belongingness. *See also* thwarted
belongingness
as basic human need, 112–13
and classroom context, 175–78
participation in affinity groups
and, 178–82
in smaller groups, 55
binge eating, 37
burnout, 105
in college, 84

call for action, 170–72
campus community, Asian
American college students'
integration into, 51–62, 64–65
campus resources, 172–74
development of, 170–72
career paths, parental expectations
and, 76–77
Centers for Disease Control and
Prevention (CDC)
data on suicides in young people
(age 10–24), 93–94
information on suicide
prevention, 91
suicide statistics, 5, 7–8

Chang, Jason Oliver, 189–90
Chang, Ying-Ying, 197–98
cheerleading, 66
Chin, Vincent, 180, 181
Chinese, as Asian Americans,
  6f, 6–7
classroom(s)
  discussions in, 177
  inclusive, creating (practice
    recommendation), 175–78
  racism in, 63–64, 175–76
classroom culture, 175–78
classroom experiences
  and good days, 134
  negative, 43–44
collectivism, and pressure for
  academic achievement, 80
college life, transition to, mental
  health challenges and, 38, 39
colleges, institutional change
  in, 170–72
college students. See also Asian
  American college students;
  research, author's,
  participants in
  global pandemic and, 15, 25–26
  mental health support for, 17, 39–
    40, 53–54
  suicidal ideation in, 5–6
  suicides among, 5–6
college students of color,
  acculturative stress in, 12–13
compassion, 26–27
  and care perspective, 141
  in narrative research, 30–31
  and self-love, 125
confidentiality, 31
cooking, and self-care,
  128–29, 166

coping
  active, 103–4
  process of, 103–4
coping strategies, 25, 27, 28f, 31–32,
  103–12, 161, 163–64
  activities used as, 105–11
coronavirus. See also COVID-19
  racialized narrative about, 189–90
counselor, as source of
  support, 117–18
COVID-19. See also pandemic
  Asian Americans blamed for,
    15–16, 62–63, 154–55, 157–58,
    180–81
  racialized narrative of, 189–90
  uncertainty and fear about, 94–99
creative projects, as coping strategy,
  108, 163–64
cultural challenges, 152–58. See also
  acculturation
  of returning home, 53–54
  roommates and, 67–69
  in transition from high school to
    college, 52–53

depression, 9–10. See also major
  depressive disorder
  in Asian American college
    students, 12, 145–46
  in middle and high school
    students, 34–40, 148–49
  pandemic and, 93–94,
    162–63
  and perceived
    burdensomeness, 22–23
  pressure for academic
    achievement and, 80
  and suicidal ideation, 11–12
Durkheim, Emile, 18–21

eating, and self-care, 128–29, 166
eating disorder, 37–38
egoistic suicide, 20
European American college
     students
  suicidal ideation in, 7–8
  suicide death rate in, 7–8
exams, stress of, 42–43
exercise
  as coping strategy, 108–10
  during pandemic, 100–1, 163
  as self-care, 126–27

faculty members
  *in loco parentis*, 145
  as representatives of campus
     culture, 175–76, 177–78
  as source of support, 113, 119
  and students, professional
     and caring relationship
     between, 175–78
family. *See also*
     intergenerational trauma
  geographic distance from, 72–73
  and perceived burdensomeness,
     22–23, 159
  as reason for living, 137–39, 168–69
  as source of support, 114–16, 117–
     19, 164–65, 182–83
  and suicide-related outcomes, 14
family bonding,
     supporting (practice
     recommendation), 182–83
family concerns, 72–73
family conflict, 45–46
family expectations, 74–75
family responsibilities, 73–74
fear, as protective factor, research
     recommendations for, 192

Filipinos, as Asian Americans,
     6f, 6–7
financial aid, 80–81
financial burden, 72, 78–80, 81,
     85, 158
financial support, 114–15
first-generation students, support
     systems for, 117–18
food
  and self-care, 128–29
  as source pleasure and pain, 37
fraternity, as source of support, 113
friends/friendships, 45–46. *See also*
     social connections
  long-term, 113
  pandemic and, 99–100
  and perceived burdensomeness,
     82–84, 159
  as protective factors, 113
  as source of support, 113, 115–20,
     165–66, 168–69
  time with, positive effects of,
     131–32, 134–35, 165–66, 168
future, promise of, as protective
     factor, 137–38, 139–43, 168, 169

generalized anxiety disorder, 40
global pandemic. *See* COVID-19;
     pandemic
good day(s), 31–32, 130–35
  accumulation of, 162, 167–68
  and bad days, balance of, 139–
     40, 167–68
  specific days as, anticipation
     of, 132–33
grades, stress related to, 84–85, 154
Greek system. *See* fraternity;
     sororities
guilt. *See* perceived burdensomeness

hate crimes, against Asian
Americans, 21. *See also* anti-
Asian incidents/hate/violence
helping professions, students'
choices of, 141–42
high school, mental health
challenges experienced in,
34–40, 148–49, 160–61
history of mental health challenges,
31–32, 34–40, 148–49
home
safety in, 88–89
students' return to, during
pandemic, 94–96, 102–3
hooks, bell, 176–78
hopelessness
in Asian American college
students, 145–46
financial and academic challenges
and, 85
in middle and high school
students, 34–40, 148–49
human attachment, 31–32, 112–
20, 161
human story(ies), 1–2, 29–32, 147. *See
also* narrative research
author's, 195–99
hydration, as self-care, 121–22, 166
hygiene
and preventing spread of COVID-
19, 97–98, 163
as self-care, 123–24, 163, 166–67

imposter syndrome, 59–61, 154
inclusive classroom. *See*
classroom(s)
Indians, as Asian Americans,
6f, 6–7
individuation, excessive, 20

*in loco parentis*, 145, 171–72
intentional activity, as self-care, 126
intergenerational conflict, 14
intergenerational trauma, 31–32, 46–
51, 148, 150–51
interpersonal expectations, 14
interviews, in narrative research, 29
invisibility, feelings of, 44, 155–56
isolation. *See also* thwarted
belongingness
of middle and high school
students, 36, 148–49
pandemic and, 15, 42, 93–
94, 162–63
at work, 44

Jamison, Kay Redfield, 197–98
Japanese, as Asian Americans,
6f, 6–7
Joiner, Thomas, 20–23, 197–98
journaling, 197
as coping strategy, 106–7, 163–64

Koreans, as Asian Americans,
6f, 6–7

liability, perceived burdensomeness
and, 22
life events, as protective factor,
research recommendations
for, 192
life skills, 26–27, 28f, 31–32, 121–29,
162, 166–67
types of, 121
loneliness, 20–21
coping strategies for, 105–11
of middle and high school
students, 36, 148–49
pandemic and, 93–94

major(s). *See also* Asian American
    Studies program
    research participants', 57, 58t
major depressive disorder, *See also*
    depression
    symptoms of, 9–10, 10b
marginalization
    of nondominant racial groups, 21
    as racial oppression, 21
Maslow, Abraham, 112–13
mass shooting, media coverage of, 8–9
May, as Mental Health Awareness
    Month, 174
meaning of life, 135–36
media coverage
    of anti-Asian hate, 16
    of Asian American college
        students' suicides, 8–9
    of mass shooting, 8–9
mental disorder. *See also* mental
    health challenges
    and perceived
        burdensomeness, 22–23
mental health, information about,
    providing to students, 172–74
Mental Health Awareness Month
    (May), 174
mental health challenges, 2. *See also*
    depression; history of mental
    health challenges; mental
    disorder
    of Asian American college
        students, 145–46
    global pandemic and, 15
    pandemic and, 93–94
    social experiences and, 12–16
mental health support, Asian
    American college students
    and, 17, 39–40, 53–54

mentors, as source of support,
    113, 119
methodology. *See also* narrative
    research
    author's, 29–32
middle school, mental health
    challenges experienced in,
    34–40, 148–49, 160–61
Midwest Asian American Students
    Union (MAASU), 180
mindfulness, 26–27, 135–36
    as coping mechanism, 111–12
    definition of, 111–12
    and self-love, 125
    and suicide resiliency, 111–12
model minority myth, 69–
    70, 154–55
moral objections, as protective
    factor, research
    recommendations for, 192
motivation, lack of, 41, 87
music
    listening to, as coping
        strategy, 105–6
    making, as coping strategy, 108

narrative(s). *See* human story(ies)
narrative research, 28, 29–32, 147. *See
    also* human story(ies); research
    participants
nature, spending time with, as
    coping strategy, 108–10
needs, Maslow's hierarchy of, 112–13
*Night Falls Fast* (Jamison), 197–98

off-campus living, social challenges
    of, 60–61
*On Earth We're Briefly Gorgeous*
    (Vuong), 46–47

ongoing suicidal thoughts, 31–32, 92, 148, 160–61
optimism, as protective factor, research recommendations for, 192
organizational change, 170–72

Pacific Islanders
    as Asian Americans, 7–8
    suicide death rates in, 19t
    U.S. Census Bureau classification of, 18
Pacific Islander students, mental health awareness programs for, 174–75
pain, psychological
    accumulation of, 33–34
    of middle and high school students, 34–40, 148–49
pandemic
    and anti-Asian incidents, 15–16
    and Asian American studies, 189–90
    and isolation, 42
    living through, and meaning/ purpose, 141
    persisting in, 2–3, 14–16, 31–32, 93–103, 147, 161, 162–63, 181–82
    psychological toll of, 93–95, 102–3, 192
    racialized narrative of, 189–90
    social effects of, 25–26
    and students' self-care, 184
    and violence, 15–16, 21
panic attack, 87, 160–61
panic disorder, 39
paradox, of vulnerability and resiliency, 8–18, 31–32, 170

parenting style, family trauma and, 48–49
parents. See also *in loco parentis*
    childhood struggles of, children's feelings about, 50, 150
    conflicts between, 45, 73–74
    conflicts with, during pandemic, 96–97
    emotional unavailability of, 48–51, 114–15, 117, 150–51, 164–65, 182–83
    gratitude to, as reason for living, 138–39
    pressures on students, 75–77
    as source of support, 114, 164–65, 182–83
    students' concerns about, during pandemic, 95–96, 163
    students' relationships with, 115, 117
parents' weekends, 182–83
perceived burdensomeness, 17, 20–23, 27, 28f, 31–32, 71–90, 148, 158–59
    among Asian American college students, 17
    definition of, 71
    and friendships, 82–84
    as risk factor, 81
perfectionism, 58–59, 80
    and suicidal ideation, 76
perpetual foreigner myth, 15–16, 68–69, 154–55, 157–58
physical activity
    as coping strategy, 108–10, 163–64
    during pandemic, 100–1, 163
    as self-care, 126–27

practice recommendations,
172–91, 193
1: create a more inclusive
classroom, 175–78
2: participate in affinity
groups, 178–82
3: support family bonding, 182–83
4: promote self-care
practices, 184–86
5: develop an Asian American
Studies major, 186–91
prayer(s), as coping strategy, 107
protective factors, 1, 23–28, 28f, 31–
32, 146–47, 164–66
characteristics of, 91–92
meaning in life as, 135–36
promotion of, 161–69
research on, recommendations
for, 192
social support as, 25–26
and suicide resilience, 91–92
types of, 91

race, and suicide death rate,
18, 19t
racial discrimination,
marginalization as, 21
racial microaggressions, 66–
67, 155–56
racism, 61–65. See also model
minority myth
Asian American college students
and, 13–14, 15–16, 61–65,
70–71, 154–58
Asian Americans' experience of,
21, 62–63
on campus, national culture and,
70–71, 181–82

in classroom, 63–64, 175–76
COVID-related, 15–16, 157–58,
180–81, 189–90 (see also
COVID-19)
indirect, 61–62
institutional, 69–70, 154–
55, 156–57
personal, 61–62
racist abuse, 67
reading
as coping strategy, 106
as self-care, 123
reasons for living, 31–32, 88, 135–43,
143t, 162, 168–69
reflection, as coping strategy,
107, 163–64
relationship conflict, 45–46, 151–52
religious affiliation, as protective
factor, 107
research recommendations
for, 192
remote learning, 94–95, 162–63
challenges of, 42
research participants
ages of, 31, 32t
majors, minors, and emphases,
57, 58t
reasons for living, 135–43,
143t, 168–69
self-care routines, 129, 130t
self-identified ethnicity of, 31, 32t
research recommendations, 191–92
resiliency. See also suicide resiliency
in children and
adolescents, 24–25
coping strategies and, 25
definition of, 23–24
elements of, 25

social support and, 25–26
against suicidal ideation, 23–25
and vulnerability, paradox of, 8–
18, 31–32, 170
resiliency theory, 27
as strengths-based
approach, 23–25
responsibility, as reason for living,
136–38, 168–69
rest, positive effects of, 131
restorying, 30–31
risk factors, 1, 27, 28, 31–32, 146–47
reducing, 147–61
for suicidal ideation, 18–23
and suicide vulnerability, 18–23
roommates
and cultural challenges, 67–
69, 157
as source of support, 113, 118–19
routine
everyday, as self-care, 122–24
during pandemic, 101–2
positive effects of, 131, 132–34
running, as coping strategy, 108–9

sadness. See perceived
burdensomeness
coping strategies for, 105–11
San Francisco State University
(SFSU), School of Ethnic
Studies, 188
schedule(s)
pandemic and, 94–95, 96, 101–2
positive effects of, 131, 132–34, 151–
52, 167–68
and self-care, 122–24
self-care, 26–27, 31–32, 121–29,
162, 166–67

campus leaders' advocacy
of, 185–86
classroom culture and, 177–78
curriculum and, 186
individual students' role
in, 184–85
pandemic and, 184
participants', 129, 130t
practices and activities of, 121–
22, 184
promotion of (practice
recommendation), 184–86
self-compassion, 26–27, 125
self-care as, 166–67
self-hate, perceived
burdensomeness and, 22
self-love, 166–67
self-reliance, 31–32, 103–12,
161, 163–64
acceptance and, 111
as coping strategy, 25
self-respect, 166–67
September, as Suicide Prevention
Month, 172–73
shame, about psychological
distress, 173–74
Shin, Elizabeth, 8–9
sibling(s)
as allies/confidants, 77, 110–11
comparisons among, 74–
75, 77–78
and preferred child status,
75–76
as reason for living, 138
as source of support, 114, 116–18,
164–65, 182–83
suicide of, author's story
of, 195–99

skin care, as self-care, 125–26,
166–67
sleep
positive effects of, 131
as self-care, 124, 166
social connections. *See also* friends/
friendships
as coping strategy, 110–11
during pandemic, 96–97,
99–100
social expectations, 152–58
in college, 56–57
social integration, 20–21, 27
social isolation, 20–21. *See also*
isolation
social support, 27, 28*f*
as protective factor, 25–26
sororities, 55, 65
as source of support, 113, 118–19
stigma, of psychological
distress, 173–74
STOP APPI Hate, 16, 62
storytelling. *See* human stories;
narrative research
stressors, for Asian American
college students, 70
student organizations. *See also*
affinity groups
formation of (creating), 179–80
importance of, 53–54, 56, 154
and regional conferences, 180
suicidal ideation. *See also* ongoing
suicidal thoughts
in Asian American college
students, 7–8, 145–46
in college students, 5–6
definition of, 4

depression and, 11–12
in European American college
students, 7–8
factors contributing to, 9–10, 14
in middle and high school
students, 34–40, 148–49
participants' descriptions of, 86–
87, 149, 160–61
perfectionism and, 76
perpetual foreigner myth
and, 68–69
and physical symptoms, 87
professional support for, among
college students, 17
resiliency against, 23–25
risk factors for, 18–23
short-versus long-term, 38–39,
148–49
and suicide deaths, 9–10
suicide. *See also* egoistic
suicide
among college students, 5–6
definition of, 4
in United States, 5–6
suicide attempt(s)
definition of, 4
participants' descriptions
of, 87–88
suicide death rate
age and, 18
in Asian American college
students, 7–9
in European American college
students, 7–8
race and, 18, 19*t*
in young people (age 18 to 24),
7–8

suicide prevention, 4, 91
Suicide Prevention Month (September), 172–73
suicide resiliency, 1–2, 18, 31–32, 161–69
  in Asian American college students, 7–8
  development of, 27–28, 28f
  mindfulness and, 111–12
  protective factors and, 23–28, 91–92
suicide vulnerability, 1, 9–17, 27–28, 28f, 31–32, 147–61
  risk factors and, 18–23
supervisors, as source of support, 119–20
support systems, 31–32, 112–20, 161. *See also* social support
  professional, 119–20
  as protective factors, 112–13, 164–66
  rule of three for, 117–19
survival, stories of, 29–30
survivor's guilt, 89

Tang, Luke, 8–9
terminology, 4–5
therapist, as source of support, 117–18
thwarted belongingness, 20–23, 27, 28f, 31–32, 51–71, 84, 148, 152–58. *See also* isolation
time management
  during pandemic, 100–1
  in pandemic, 162–63
  as self-care, 125

transgender Asian American college students, research on, recommendations for, 192
trauma. *See also* intergenerational trauma; racial microaggressions
  racial, 21

United States, suicides in, 5–6
universities, institutional change in, 170–72
University of California, Berkeley (UCB), Ethnic Studies Department, 188
Urtula, Alexander, 8–9
U.S. Census Bureau, classifications of Asian Americans, 18

Vietnamese, as Asian Americans, 6f, 6–7
violence
  anti-Asian, 181–82 (*see also* anti-Asian incidents/hate/violence)
  Asian American college students and, 13–14
  in the home, 49–50
  pandemic and, 15–16, 21
vulnerability. *See also* suicide vulnerability
  and resiliency, paradox of, 8–18, 31–32, 170

walking
  as coping strategy, 108–10, 163
  during pandemic, 100–1

workouts. *See* exercise

yoga
  as coping strategy, 108–9,
    163–64
  as self-care, 127
Young, Iris, 21

young people (age 18 to 24). *See also*
    college students
  depression in, 93–94
  mental health of, pandemic
    and, 93–94
  suicide death rate in, 7–8, 18, 93–94
  suicides among, 5–6